Bela Banerjee
Bringing Health To
India's Villages

Bela Banerjee
Bringing Health To India's Villages

LaVonne Godwin Platt

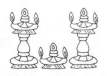

WORDSWORTH
Newton, Kansas

Credits:
Part 1—Used by permission of Macmillan Publishing Company, New York, and Unwin Hyman Ltd., London: *The Religion of Man* By Rabindranath Tagore (New York: Macmillan, 1931)

Part 2—Used by permission of Macmillan Publishing Company, New York, and Macmillan Publishers Ltd., London: "Fruit-Gathering XXXI" in *Collected Poems and Plays of Rabindranath Tagore*, (London: Macmillan, 1936, 1955, and New York: Copyright 1916 by Macmillan Publishing Company, renewed 1944 by Rabindranath Tagore)

Part 3—Used by permission of Macmillan Publishers Ltd., London: from "Gitanjali" in *Collected Poems and Plays of Rabindranath Tagore*, (London: Macmillan, 1936, 1955)

Part 4—Used by permission of Macmillan Publishing Company, New York and Macmillan Publishers Ltd., London: from *Fireflies* by Rabindranath Tagore (New York: Macmillan, 1928, renewed by Rabindranath Tagore, 1955)

Part 5—Used by permission of Macmillan Publishers Ltd., London: from "Gitanjali" in *Collected Poems and Plays of Rabindranath Tagore*, (London: Macmillan, 1936, 1955)

Part 6—Used by permission of Macmillan Publishing Company, New York and Macmillan Publishers Ltd., London: from *Fireflies* by Rabindranath Tagore (New York: Macmillan, 1928, renewed by Rabindranath Tagore, 1955)

Part 7—Used by permission of Macmillan Publishing Company, New York and Macmillan Publishers Ltd., London: from *Fireflies* by Rabindranath Tagore (New York: Macmillan, 1928, renewed by Rabindranath Tagore, 1955)

Part 8—Used by permission of Macmillan Publishers Ltd., London: from "Gitanjali" in *Collected Poems and Plays of Rabindranath Tagore*, (London: Macmillan, 1936, 1955)

Design credits: Kamala Platt; Gary Gaeddert of Asla, Gaeddert & Lee, Newton, Kansas; John Hiebert

Photo credits: David Bassett, Joan Court, Olive Grabham, Louis Grisoglio, Dipankar Nigoyin, Caroline Balderston Parry, Deborah Vaughan, Roscoe Warren, Huston Westover, Kermit Whitehead, Mike Wood.

For all those whose lives have been touched by Bela Banerjee

ACKNOWLEDGMENTS

This book was made possible through the help of many people. The Educational Foundation Program of the American Association of University Women awarded me an Individual Member Research and Project Grant in 1982-83 that helped to fund the initial research. In 1984-85 they assisted with an additional Research and Project Grant to help meet expenses involved in collecting photographic material for the book. A Friends Medical Society contribution helped meet other expenses, as did contributions by some of Bela's friends and other people who came to know about her. For this financial help and the interest in this project that it represented, I am deeply grateful.

It is difficult to decide whose names to include in this list of acknowledgments. Through taped interviews, letters, telephone conversations, and visits, more than 200 people have had a part in this telling of Bela Banerjee's story. At least a dozen people have given me guidance in the research process and in putting the manuscript together. Scores of people who heard something of Bela's story for the first time have responded with enthusiasm, encouraging me to make the written story available to them. Twelve families or village projects hosted Bela and me when we traveled together in India. I haven't counted the number of meals I had in the homes of Bela's friends and relatives in India, England, and the U.S., as I gathered research to tell her story, but they were many, and all of them included good food and good fellowship. Those readers who fall into any of the above categories, please know that I appreciate greatly what you have done to make this book possible. For special help and encouragment I thank Dr. David Bassett, Elise Boulding, Hetty Budgen, Olive Grabham, Anna Glazebrook, Lorraine K. Cleveland, Sati and Bhupendranath Ghose, Dr. Balabhadra and Kanaka Mahapatra, Kamala and Indubhushan Misra, Dr. Dhirendranath and Saki Mund, John G. Sommer, Marjorie Sykes, Deborah Vaughan and Dr. Huston and Jane Westover. Among those who provided helpful advice in manuscript preparation were Jill Benedict, Susan Janzen, Dwight Krehbiel, Marion Preheim, and Muriel Stackley. I want especially to thank my family—Dwight, Kamala, and Richard—whose encouragement, guidance, and support sustained me throughout this project.

CONTENTS

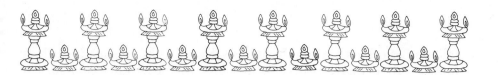

PREFACE

Countless women through the centuries have made creative differences within the context of their own cultures while remaining nameless to the larger world. Bela Banerjee is such a woman. Bela has been a positive influence in the lives of thousands of people in India. Her work not only improved health standards in remote areas of her homeland, but it also increased the acceptance of women in leadership roles in the villages where, for three decades, she trained village women to be health workers.

Laksmi Menon, who served on the United Nations Commission on the Status of Women has said that Bela Banerjee is one of the women who make a difference in India. "People who work quietly, side by side among those whom they want to raise up, are doing the hardest work, and it is generally unsung and unrecognized," Laksmi Menon said. "Bela is one of hundreds of women in India who have suffered and sacrificed to bring relief to others, never craving for power or position for themselves."

Bela Banerjee is not famous, even within India, except in places where she has worked. In those places the attitudes toward her range from reverence to friendly rapport. When she meets villagers whom she knew years before, some whisper her name in awe and bow down to touch her feet, reminding her about their baby whose life she saved at birth—or a child she nursed through a long illness. Others shout with joy when they recognize her and come running, eager to say that because of her they drink well water instead of water from the pond—or that the latrine she persuaded them to install years before has been moved to the new house they built.

Marjorie Sykes, who helped develop the basic education program at the Gandhian ashram of Sevagram and was an adviser to Quaker projects where Bela worked, described Bela's unique relationships with people. "Bela is just an average human being, like millions and millions of others," Marjorie Sykes said. "Yet she has made such an impact on so many people who were, in the world's standard of measurement, much more important and much more prominent, academic or intellectual than she." Even more important, Marjorie said, "is the impact she has made on all the people who can't talk, who have no voice, because they are illiterate and without influence."

As a child Bela Banerjee lived in a half-brother's Calcutta home where she helped her widowed mother do the cooking and manage the household. Attending school was not an option for her circumscribed life. Nonetheless, she possessed an inquiring mind which helped her learn to read and write Bengali, and later, English.

During adolescence she began to work with the Bengal Social Service League. Over a ten-year period, she was matron at their women's hostel and assistant in the orphanage and maternal and child health clinic.

Soon after the end of World War II, she joined British and American Quakers in Calcutta to be a midwife on their health team. Her sensitivity to the needs of women and children, coupled with her outreaching personality, inspired members of the Calcutta Friends Unit to arrange a scholarship for her to study nursing in London.

Upon returning to India, Bela trained young village women to provide maternal and child health care in their communities. First associated with the American Friends Service Committee's ten-year Barpali Village Service project in Orissa, she has worked for more than 30 years both in internationally staffed, large-scale village development projects and in small, indigenous social service projects. She and the scores of village health workers whom she trained helped to change village people's expectations of health care for themselves and their children and to broaden their acceptance of health professions as proper vocations for young women.

Bela Banerjee combines thorough training with a grass-roots approach. "She applies advanced western nursing techniques to ordinary people and their ordinary needs in villages," a person acquainted with her work over the years told me.

Another spoke of Bela's combination of "enthusiasm about her work and a warmth of personality that radiates friendliness to everybody." Those who worked with Bela knew that they "could rely on her to be there, to notice what people needed, or what jobs needed to be done."

Ralph Victor, an American doctor with whom Bela worked in a village development project, was struck by the fact that "Bela was what she did rather than a personality separate from her devoted work. She functioned not only as a nurse but as a healer," he said.

Wherever she is, Bela identifies with other people. "She is like a sister to us," one co-worker said. "Like a mother," said village girls she trained to be health workers. More than one villager who had been her patient told me, "When Bela comes to my house, she has come to her own house."

People who came in contact with her on her study trips to England and the United States recognized a similar bond. One of my neighbors in Kansas expressed a sentiment shared by many others when she said, "When I first met Bela, I felt as though I had known her all my life." Almost universally, an immediate closeness develops between Bela and the people she encounters. Perhaps it is because, as Roderick Ede (long-time leader in the British Friends Council) put it, "Bela is absolutely natural with everybody and expects them to be with her."

In many ways Bela Banerjee has not changed much since the mid-1950s when she and I both worked at Barpali Village Service. My first impressions of her as an effective agent of change—whether she was treating patients, delivering babies, teaching health workers, or visiting with villagers—were substantiated whenever I met her later, on short visits both in India and the United States.

To learn more of Bela's story I spent nearly six weeks with her in 1982. We traveled together by train, bus, taxi, car, jeep, cycle rickshaw, and on foot to interview family members, friends, and co-workers. We went from West Bengal to Orissa, Kerala, and Madhya Pradesh, visiting four places where she had worked in the past and two projects to which she was then affiliated as *pratinidhi* (administrator) of the Orissa section of the Kasturba Gandhi National Memorial Trust.

Bela started out speaking her native Bengali, but switched readily to Malayalam, Hindi, or Oriya, depending on whether we were in the crowded streets of Calcutta, the mountains of Kerala, the plains of Madhya Pradesh, or the rolling uplands of Orissa. Each conversation she translated in English, so that I could understand. Not fluent in any of the languages except Bengali, she communicated well in all of them.

As we traveled, we talked about the next place we would visit. Before we reached each destination, Bela described the project, her co-workers there, and the villagers she had known. She reflected on her experiences in the area and told me about the changes that she had observed on her last visit. She speculated about whom we would be likely to see and mentioned some who had died or moved away since she had left.

Bela's excitement mounted whenever the landscape became familiar to her. Each time as we neared our destination, her anticipation became contagious. When we were scheduled to reach the village of Barpali in Orissa, we were both so eager that we moved our luggage down the aisle of the train a full 20 minutes before arrival time and stood peering out the doorway like the ticketless travelers preparing to jump off before reaching the station platform.

After almost constant activity in the places where everyone knew Bela, we relaxed in the Orissa town of Burla where she had never lived. There we visited Dr. Balabhadra Mahapatra and his wife Kanaka, with whom Bela had worked 30 years before at Barpali.

One evening Bela, Kanaka, and I were sitting on a *charpoy* (a village cot of woven rope on a wooden frame) in the courtyard of the Mahapatra home, leisurely visiting. I watched the change of color on a patch of marigolds as the sun neared the horizon, but my mind was still on the interviews I had had with the Mahapatras earlier in the day.

Kanaka must have been thinking about our conversation, too, and wanting to share some of it with Bela. She turned to her and said in Oriya, "Bela, you were born poor and you are still poor, but you have traveled all over the world and have had opportunities that most people with much money have never had. You are not an official, you are not rich, but you have friends all over the world. You never studied in school, but you know six languages. You have no home, but God has blessed you with many friends who count you as one of their family."

In those words, Kanaka Mahapatra had captured some of the essence of Bela Banerjee's life. Always Bela has balanced the contentment she has felt in each opportunity to serve others with a vision of a better life for those with whom she identified. Having caught "the vision of life and of love" described by the poet Rabindranath Tagore, Bela Banerjee changed her world—for herself and those around her—as she brought health to India's villages.

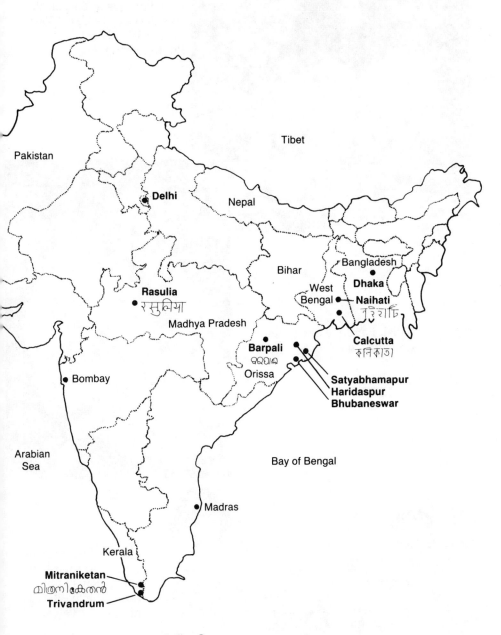

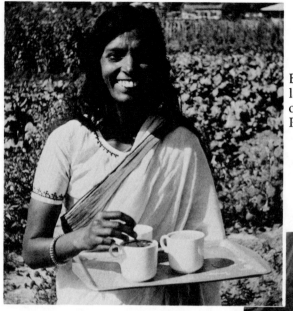

Bela Banerjee at Barpali Village Service, 1956. (© Westover of Woodstock Photography)

Satish Banerjee at his home in Calcutta, mid-1960s.

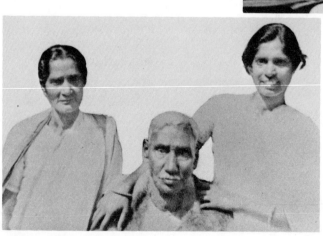

Bela, her sister Sushama, and their half-brother Satish with whom she lived as a child, early 1940s.

PART ONE:

CHILDHOOD IN AN EXTENDED FAMILY

The eternal Dream
*   is borne on the wings of ageless Light*
*   that rends the veil of the vague*
*   and goes across Time*
*   weaving ceaseless patterns of Being.*
The mystery remains dumb,
*   the meaning of this pilgrimage,*
*   the endless adventure of existence—*
whose rush along the sky
*   flames up into innumerable rings of paths,*
till at last knowledge gleams out from the dusk
*   in the infinity of human spirit,*
*   and in that dim lighted dawn*
*   she speechlessly gazes through the break in*
*   the mist*
*   at the vision of Life and Love*
rising from the tumult of profound pain and joy.

—Rabindranath Tagore,
from *The Religion of Man*

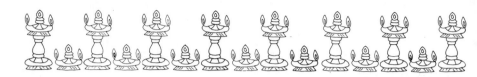

1
A VILLAGE BEGINNING

Bela had told me about the child Tankamoni while we were on the long train trip from Orissa to Kerala to visit the health center at the Mitraniketan village development project. Now, as we walked toward the little girl who stood waiting at the fork of the path, Bela hesitated. Was this child really Tankamoni? Many things were unchanged in the two years since Bela had last visited Mitraniketan, but children grow, lose teeth, and cut their hair.

"Tankamoni?" Bela called out. The child smiled bashfully but did not answer. Puzzled, Bela turned to Shanta, the health worker who was our hostess. Shanta nodded her head.

Laughing now, Bela hurried down the path to the little girl. Tankamoni waited until Bela came close. Then shyness overcame her, and she turned and ran up the hill to her home.

"She's going to get her mother," Bela guessed, and we went on with Shanta to the hospitality room where we were to stay.

An hour later Tankamoni and her mother arrived at our room. The little girl had changed from play shorts to a full-skirted, knee-length, white dress of nylon organdy—"her dancing dress," said her mother in Malayalam, the language of Kerala. She had put on silver ankle bracelets and brightly-colored glass bangles, but when Bela asked her to dance and sing, she was too timid to perform.

"She is so pretty," Bela said, addressing me but looking at the child. "She was very pretty when she was little, too," she added, smiling as she reminisced.

As the story unfolded, however, it was clear that no one had ever suggested that Tankamoni was pretty when her mother first brought her to Mitraniketan. Then she had been a malnourished six-month-old baby, with bloated abdomen and wasted limbs, lying limp in her mother's arms. Tankamoni's mother, rejected by her parents because she had given birth to an illegitimate baby, had come to the Mitraniketan project for help.

Bela had taken the young mother and her baby into the Mitraniketan health center to live with her and the health workers. She started treating the baby for protein-calorie deficiency. "We gave food. Just food. No medicine I gave," she said, describing the regimen. At first she had supplemented the inadequate supply of the mother's breast milk with cows' milk from the Mitraniketan dairy. After a few days she added mashed carrots mixed with milk and, later, semolina, a wheat cereal. Finally she fed Tankamoni mashed carrots, potatoes, beans, and *dhal* (lentils) mixed with egg.

During the first days Bela made the mixture and fed the baby herself, demonstrating to the health workers how to give her small amounts at each feeding, several times a day. Then she showed Tankamoni's mother how to prepare and apportion the feedings.

Bela's tenderness toward Tankamoni ran deeper than knowing that she had saved the child's life. "Whenever I see that kind of malnutrition in babies I think to myself, I used to be like that," Bela said.

Bela Banerjee was born near the Bengali city of Dhaka, in the village of Butani, to Mukunda Chandra Banerjee, a schoolmaster, and his third wife Bimula. Guesses at the year of her birth vary from 1913 to 1919.

In addition to her brother Monesh and her sister Sushama, Bela had two half brothers Satish and Gan, and a half sister Hamonta, children of Mukunda Banerjee's first two wives, who had both died of cholera. Gan, the second wife's son, lived with Bela's family in the village. Satish, the older half brother, and his sister Hamonta were both married and lived with their families in Calcutta.

When Bela was about seven months old, her father died, also of cholera. Because of a village superstition that the recent birth of a baby may cause a parent to die, Bela was blamed for Mukunda Banerjee's death. Bimula Banerjee, believing the superstition and despondent over her husband's death, stopped feeding Bela or taking care of her other needs. By the time the neglect became obvious, Bela was severely malnourished.

At that point an elderly servant named Joydeb took it upon himself to feed Bela and to care for her whenever she was left alone. Because he was a Harijan, an untouchable, Joydeb was not allowed to cook in the Brahman household of the Banerjees, but each day after Bela's mother had fed Monesh, Sushama, and Gan, Joydeb would feed Bela something that was left.

Bela's aunt, who lived in a separate household in the same compound, helped Joydeb by giving maternal care to the neglected baby. Bela soon became a favorite of her aunt, who had two sons but no daughters.

Even after her time of mourning had passed, Bimula Banerjee found it difficult to provide for her children. The problem was most evident in financial matters. Although the family owned property from which they received income, she did not manage it well. Other relatives took advantage of her financial ineptitude.

Eventually, with little money remaining, Bimula Banerjee took Bela and Sushama to live with her brothers in the town of Khilgaon, a suburb of Dhaka, where earlier she had sent Monesh so that he could attend school. Before long, Bimula's brothers said they could not continue to take care of her and her children. She decided to go to live with Satish, her older stepson.

Bimula Banerjee must have known that she and her children might not be eagerly welcomed when they came to make their home with Satish. In the first place, Satish had a family of eight children to support on his salary as a journalist. It would not be easy for him to suddenly increase his responsibilities to include another family of four.

The situation might have been even more difficult, had Satish not possessed a generous, forgiving nature. Years before, while attending college in Calcutta, Satish had joined the Brahmo Samaj, a religious reform movement that rejected the Hindu practices of caste discrimination and idol worship. Although Mukunda Banerjee had also been active in the Brahmo Samaj in his home district, where the organization was still tied to traditional Hinduism, he could not accept the progressive ideas of his son Satish and other young intellectuals who broke completely from Hindu practices.

When Satish had discarded the sacred thread that designated his Brahman manhood, Mukunda Banerjee refused to accept his son's break with the traditional society and told Satish he was no longer welcome at his parental home. Eventually Satish and his father were reconciled, but Satish's children grew up feeling the effects of the years of separation from their grandfather and the extended family to which they belonged.

Into these circumstances Bimula Banerjee brought her three children in the mid-1920s, when Bela was probably eight or ten years old. At the time, Satish's family was living in Madhupur, one of several towns in Bihar to which they moved from time to time to get away from what Satish considered the unhealthful air in Calcutta. Whenever the family lived in Bihar, Satish rented a room for himself in a boarding house in Calcutta, where his work was located, and commuted by train to be with his family on weekends.

Bimula had written to Satish that she and her children were coming; Satish met their train in Calcutta and accompanied them to Madhupur. At the Madhupur train station they transferred their belongings to a *tonga*, a horse-drawn carriage, which took them to the home where Satish's wife and children were waiting.

When the *tonga* arrived at the Banerjee door, bringing their father with four strangers—three of them children peering around the carriage sides—Satish's children knew that an abrupt change was about to occur in their family structure. Samiran Banerjee, Satish's second son, reminisced about that day when I met him at his home in England, where he is a psychiatrist. Even though his parents had agreed to accept Bimula and her children into their home, Samiran remembered that they were worried about the financial strain of adding more people to their already large family. They were also concerned about the new pattern of family life that would need to be developed to accommodate the relatives who had come to live with them.

Samiran talked about the tension his family had felt. But more importantly, he recalled that it was alleviated when Bela's family arrived. "What I observed," Samiran said, "was that when Bishima (he referred to Bela as Bishima, a Bengali word meaning aunt) got down from the *tonga*, she came with a big smile. She looked around and kept on smiling, and the tenseness in the situation subsided."

"Perhaps I am philosophizing," Samiran admitted, as he related the story to me, "but I did notice these things. I thought that here is a person who is so sensitive and perceptive, there will be no problem. That was the first impression I had, and it continued." According to Samiran the tension which had affected everyone in his family was replaced by a friendly relationship that developed between the two families. "And Bishima was the pivot around which it grew," he said. "Always she was smiling and giving what we wanted—before we asked her for anything, she was there with it."

Bela's good nature alone could not account for the lessening of the tensions between the two families. Her mother also promoted a better relationship when she proposed that she and her two daughters do the household work in exchange for Satish providing a home for her and her children and an opportunity for Monesh to continue his education.

Satish agreed, letting go nearly all the servants except those who did the heavy work and that which Bela's mother could not do because of Brahman caste restrictions.

As a member of the Brahmo Samaj, Satish did not agree with the Hindu restrictions that set the pattern of life for Brahman widows. Nevertheless, he arranged for his stepmother to have the separate pots, pans, and *chula* (stove) for her cooking fire that she believed necessary. She ate only one meal a day—usually rice and potatoes—and that not until after she had finished cooking and serving food to the others. Sometimes, because of her responsibilities in managing Satish's household, she did not start her own meal preparation until after ten o'clock at night.

Overly cautious about spending money unnecessarily with Satish providing for her, Bela's mother purchased neither soap for her bath nor oil for her hair. She had similar concern about the use of her time. Because it took extra time to comb her long hair, she cut it.

Again and again she reminded her children about Satish's generosity. "Because of Satish, we could come here and stay. Otherwise, I don't know what we would have done," she would say to Bela, as they worked together around the house. "God has helped us all so well."

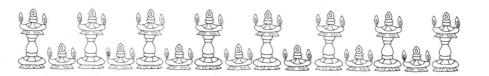

2
WORK AND STUDY IN SATISH'S HOME

In the waiting room of the Madras train station, Bela Banerjee bathed and changed her *sari*, replacing the long cloth, limp from being worn two nights and a day on the train, with another that was crisply starched and ironed. Both *saris* were homespun, differing only in the fineness of the weave and the color and design of the border on the otherwise white expanse of cotton fabric. She combed her freshly shampooed black hair, beginning to gray, and, favoring her arthritic left arm, asked another woman to twist her hair into a bun just above the nape of her neck.

Back on the train to continue our journey to the places where she had lived and worked, Bela talked to me about her life. More than a week on the trains provided ample time for visiting, as we traveled down the eastern coast from Calcutta to Bhubaneswar and then to Madras, west to the Kerala coastal city of Trivandrum, north to Hoshangabad in Madhya Pradesh, and southeast to villages in Orissa.

At night our reservations on the second class sleeper gave each of us the right to one of three tiers of the flat board sleeping accommodations on either side of a narrow compartment. Our compartment opened onto an aisle that ran along one side of the train car, connecting a row of similar compartments. During the day the middle berths were lowered against the wall, transforming each bottom berth to seating designed for three passengers. Frequently, instead of three, the benches held six or seven people crowded together, especially when daytime passengers who did not require reservations boarded the train. Beneath the windows across the side aisle were single seats, facing one another in pairs; they, too, could be made into berths at night.

We got acquainted in an informal fashion with our compartment companions: the young college student on his way home for the *Durga Puja* holidays (a religious celebration) who wanted to know why I was always writing in my notebook; the older businessman who recommended his favorite books to help me "understand the real India"; the three-generation joint family who moved in with large baskets of food and promptly set up housekeeping in what appeared to be an attempt to eat their way across the country, perhaps to keep the children occupied.

Hour after hour we traveled past thatched-roof earthen houses clustered together in villages surrounded by green rice fields reaching to tree-covered hills along the horizon. Beside each village were ponds where people bathed, washed their clothes, and watered their cattle. Occasionally ducks swam on the surface of the ponds. Egrets fed on insects along the banks or perched on the backs of the cows. The scene varied from day to day as backwater bays lined with palm trees, pineapple, and tapioca in southwestern India gave way to orange trees, mustard plants and scrub jungle in the dry central plains. In each part of the country the landscape was as I remembered it 25 years before; it was easy to visualize an even earlier time that Bela talked about when she described her childhood in her half brother's home.

"At first I was quite small, so I only helped my sister and my mother prepare the meals," Bela said, telling of her responsibilities in Satish's home. "After my sister was married, I learned to cook."

"Only helping," as Bela described her duties, consisted of grinding spices, washing and cutting up vegetables, rolling out *chappaties*, and serving food to Satish and his family and her brother Monesh. They sat on bamboo mats and ate from brass plates, deftly rolling the rice and vegetables into small portions to eat with their fingers. Following the traditional pattern of serving meals in Indian families, Bela and her sister Sushama ate after the others had eaten.

When she was small, Bela was given an occasional break from the housework. Then she and Shefalika, the niece closest in age to her, would play house, using small stones and chips of clay tile instead of dolls.

When they lived in Bihar, the two little girls sometimes went with older members of the family to the market. "I was interested in the bangles," Bela said, describing the brightly colored glass bracelets that Indian women and girls wear in sets of four or more on each arm. "And I liked to look at the tribal people who came there. I liked the blouses and other clothes that the tribal women wore."

As she grew older, sometimes Bela would join her nieces and nephews in a card game they called Twenty-one. "Caroms I also used to play with them, although I was not very good at it," she remembered. It was the camaraderie that she enjoyed. "My nieces and nephews were quite friendly, and we used to talk and laugh together."

The train stopped in a station. "*Chai, chai* (Tea, tea)," the vendors called out, passing beneath the train windows. We ordered some, and the *chai walla* poured it steaming hot from his kettle, milk and sugar already added. He handed the cups to us between the horizontal bars of the open window.

I thought of recent mornings when we were guests in friends' homes; each day as we wakened, someone from the family had brought us cups of tea. That reminded me of Bela's childhood responsibilities. "Did you serve tea to all of Satish's family every day before breakfast?" I asked.

"No," Bela said, "nobody had tea except Satish. When he was at home, I usually made his tea and served it to him before he had breakfast." She sipped her own tea and smiled, as though she was remembering a pleasant break in her early morning routine.

In Satish's home Bela's day began at 5:00 or 5:30. Before anyone else was up, she and her sister and mother started the cooking fire to prepare Satish's tea and to cook breakfast. "In Bihar we used a smoky coal for our fuel. We would burn it first and then cook over the hot coals," Bela explained. "When we lived in Calcutta, we had better coal that didn't smoke; we could cook right on it."

The source of water was different in the two locations as well. In Calcutta water came from taps in the courtyard. In Bihar a man was hired to carry it into the house from a nearby well.

After finishing her breakfast duties, Bela's next job each day was to prepare lunch for her nieces and nephews to take to school. She packed each lunch of *chappaties* and a dry curry of potatoes or lentils into a "tiffin box"—a round tin with a tight-fitting lid.

At 4:00 in the afternoon, and again at 10:00 in the night, Bela's nieces and nephews and her brothers began to arrive for the main meals of rice and dhal and at least two curries. "Whenever they liked to eat, they came in," Bela remembered. In between, she told me, she kept the food warm and the eating area clean. "That was going on until 12:00 o'clock. Then I finished cleaning up—covering and clearing and closing everything. Time by then was always 12:30 or 1:00."

Bela's nephews and nieces remembered, too. "We were a bit careless," Samiran said. "After our study and after games and things, we used to come for our meals—not all at once, but one by one—making a lot of trouble for her."

Samiran continued. "She had a hard life, but she never complained. She never said, 'Oh, why are you not coming all at one time?'"

When no one was eating, Bela studied. And when she was too tired, she put three or four low wooden seats together and lay down to rest. Samiran remembered that when someone would come into the room, she would raise up—"Oh, who is there?" she would ask— and she would get up and serve their meal.

"We took advantage of her, and nobody told us not to," Samiran said.

Bela did not complain, even to herself. "That's the way I learned to cook and to take care of things," she told me. "I could manage everything very well."

Bela also helped her mother with the housework. "Every day we had a lot of cleaning to do—and washing clothes and ironing—it was a big house, and my mother was a very, very clean person," she said.

"Didn't you sometimes feel tired?" I asked her.

"No, I didn't feel I was very tired."

I persisted. "Weren't there times when you didn't want to do all those things?"

"No, I never felt like that," she insisted. "I always felt that was my job; that's the way I'm going to live. And I was quite happy."

Bela, like her mother, appreciated the opportunity to work and live in Satish's home. Extremely devoted to her half brother, she accepted for herself the selflessness that she saw in him. When a friend in Calcutta talked about Bela's constant work from morning to night, Bela interrupted. "I did it for my nieces and nephews," she said. "That's why I'm very fond of them."

When the nieces and nephews helped with small household chores, Bela was adept at organizing the duties, matching each person to the right job. Samiran told me that even though Bela was younger than most of them, "she managed so well that everyone was satisfied."

One of her nieces described Bela's managerial skills with less generosity. "I was afraid of her and thought that I had to do what she said." She laughed, telling about being called to meals or to do some work, when she wanted to continue playing or reading.

From her mother, Bela gleaned a sense of economy. She would notice if a light was on and nobody was in the room and she would turn the light off. "The household ran much better when she and her elder sister and their mother took over the management," a nephew remembered.

After Bela's sister was married, Kripa, Satish's wife, helped with more of the work. Bela enjoyed those times when Kripa and she worked together around the house. "My sister-in-law used to sing," Bela remembered. "While she was sweeping and dusting, she was singing. In the early afternoon when everyone had finished eating, she would come through the room to sweep, and she would sing a Brahmo Samaj song. I still have that song in my ear—she used to sing like that." Malay, Bela's oldest nephew, said that Bela also sang as she worked, having learned the Brahmo Samaj songs from his mother.

Bela's desire to please Kripa caused her to work very hard; usually she was rewarded with the affection she sought. Somewhat afraid of her sister-in-law, however, she became upset whenever Kripa scolded her. If Kripa said that the food tasted greasy or over-seasoned, for example, Bela would refuse to eat. Then Kripa would console her with a kiss and make it a point to tell others, "I wish I had one daughter like Bela."

Kripa was an important influence in Bela's life. "Her scolding sometimes made me cry, but I think it made me more independent also," Bela told me.

Education was important to the Banerjee family. All eight of Satish's children finished high school and six of them graduated from college, one of them continuing his education through medical school. Bela's brother Monesh studied dentistry. Even Bela's sister Sushama had attended primary school in the village before they came to live with Satish.

Bela was seven or eight years younger than her sister, and when they left their village home she had never gone to school. Because the arrangement to live in Satish's home did not include educational opportunities for her and her sister, Bela did not attend school at all when she was a child.

Although Bela's mother had received little schooling, she was literate and could read the Hindu scriptures, the *Bhagavad Gita*, most of which she had memorized. Sometimes when they had a few spare moments from household chores, or late at night after the work was done, she showed Bela how to write simple sentences in Bengali. "My mother did not know how to do good writing," Bela said, "and I, too, still cannot write correctly." She laughed at what she considered to be her own ineptitude.

Some of Satish's children had most of their education at home with tutors until they completed secondary school and entered the university. Others went to Christian mission schools or to the poet Rabindranath Tagore's ashram at Santiniketan.

"In our home was lots of education," Bela said. "All my nieces and nephews were studying, so I was interested." Sometimes she managed to be working in the room where her nieces and nephews had classes with the tutor, so that she could listen. "I was busy with the housework, but my ear was always hearing what they were learning, so it helped me a lot. Even when I was working at the housework and cooking, I would stop sometimes and do some handwriting or read a little in a book that was nearby. When I had some free time in the afternoon I would sit with my nieces Jutika and Shefalika when they were studying, and whatever they were writing, I would copy," she added.

I wondered if Bela didn't wish she could go along with her nieces when they went to school, but she seemed not to have thought about it. "I wished I could learn more—that is true—but I was so happy with my work that I was not really thinking very much that I should go and study. I was more involved with my work and doing that right. My mind was always occupied with the job I was doing. I never felt jealous because they were going to school and I was not.

"Whatever I was doing, I felt that those were the things I should do. Actually my mind was never that I would ever go away from that house. I will be there all my life—that was my thought."

Kripa Banerjee sometimes gave lessons to Bela along with her own children. "She was a very good teacher," Bela said. "I liked her way of explaining Bengali poems." Picking up her education from her nieces and nephews as they studied with their mother, Bela learned about Rabindranath Tagore, whose poetry was very popular in Calcutta at the time.

"One Tagore poem my sister-in-law used to read was about a man who was searching for a god and went to all the holy places but could not find the god. When he came home he found it in his hand." Bela paused, and I thought how such a philosophy allowed her to be satisfied with her restricted life even though she had a vision of a wider world in her dreams.

"My sister-in-law explained that story so beautifully the first time I heard it," Bela said. Tagore's poems influenced Bela greatly. "Tagore came from a wealthy family, but he knew the life of the poor people so well," she said. "What really happens, he knew. When you read a Tagore poem, you feel like you are in that place," she continued. "Tagore wrote beautiful poetry about the rivers of India and about little things."

She was particularly attracted to a Tagore poem with the theme, "I didn't do what I said I would do." Bela looked up at me as she spoke. "I've thought about that poem a lot in my life.

"There were other stories that my sister-in-law told and beautiful songs that she sang from the Brahmo Samaj hymnal." Bela continued. "And all these things made my insides different."

Bela looked at me again, her eyes questioning whether I knew what she meant. I nodded, and she went on to describe Brahmo Samaj beliefs. Without criticizing Hinduism, which she also respected, she compared the two faiths. "Brahmo Samaj worship is different from Hindu worship," she said. "In Hindu worship you make an idol, give flowers, and burn incense. Brahmo Samaj idea is a deep feeling. Especially their beautiful songs—and the meanings of the songs. I used to listen to the songs and think that this was really true—the idea that people are the most important. It is always in my mind to be friendly and to be with the people."

She applied the same philosophy to her work in village development. "I like to know the people instead of going to conferences and listening to big lectures," she said. "I think that mixing with the people is more important than giving speeches. I go to a house to visit. I am with them—one of them—I have come to see some friends. Like that I like to work. It comes from in the heart, really."

Considering the ideas that she pondered and the values that she incorporated into her life while still a child, who is to say that Bela did not receive an education in Satish's home?

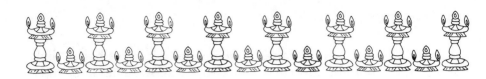

3
A FAMILY TRADITION OF SIMPLICITY

An American doctor who met Bela Banerjee when she was on a study tour in the United States in 1963 went to India for a family planning conference some years later. Upon arriving in Calcutta and remembering that Bela's brother lived there, the doctor decided to telephone him and ask about Bela. He could not remember Satish's name, but thought that he would recall it when he looked at the Banerjee names in the telephone directory. Opening the phone book to the first Banerjee, his eyes scanned column after column of the Banerjee name. He turned the page. More Banerjees. Page after page of Banerjees. And following that spelling of the name were other variations in the English translation.

The doctor had not known that Banerjee is among the most common Bengali family names. Derived from the ancient name of Bandyopaohyay, its roots are shared with the Tagore family that produced the poet Rabindranath, and earlier his father Debendranath, a 19th century leader of the Brahmo Samaj religious reform movement.

The branch of the Banerjee family to which Bela belongs follows a particular pattern of simplicity that Malay Banerjee called "the quality of nonattachment to property." Malay, the oldest son of Bela's half brother Satish, told me that Bela's self-giving lifestyle embodies that simplicity. "She has that characteristic of our family," he said, explaining that Bela gives little importance to material possessions or affluence. To illustrate the family tradition, Malay told about his great-grandfather, Bela's grandfather, Ram Chandra Banerjee.

The story Malay told began with Ram Chandra Banerjee as a young man, walking along the road beside the River Ganges on his way to the holy city of Benares. Although he belonged to a wealthy family of large landholders, Ram Chandra was not going to Benares to conduct family business. Quite the contrary. Ram Chandra was going to the holy city because he had decided to withdraw from the worldly affairs of the *zamindar* (landlord) system in which his family had collected revenue for the British in exchange for control of large tracts of land farmed by peasants. In Benares he hoped to find a *guru*, a teacher, to lead him in the life of an ascetic.

How did it happen that Ram Chandra, a young *zamindar* at the beginning of his career, should choose to take on the role of an ascetic? Ram Chandra's family was one of several *zamindar* families in the area whose disputes over land had frequently erupted into bloodshed. With practically no governmental control over land ownership, anybody who was powerful enough could grab the land and other property of neighboring *zamindars*. Having already been widowed when his child-bride had died, it was almost more than Ram Chandra could bear when one of his sisters was killed in an encounter with another *zamindar* family. Because of his sister's death, Ram Chandra made a vow to renounce his inherited role as a *zamindar*.

Leaving his father's ancestral village of Belghoria, he set out alone on the long pilgrimage to Benares, where he hoped to find new direction for his life. One day, as he stopped along the riverbank to cook his food, two Brahman women drew their boat up to the shore nearby. Observing the sacred thread that hung over Ram Chandra's shoulder, the women knew that the young man also was a Brahman, and they invited him into their boat to continue the trip up the Ganges. Eager to reach Benares, Ram Chandra accepted.

"Why are you going to Benares?" one of the women asked.

"I have an aversion to worldly affairs," Ram Chandra replied. "I was married and my wife died, and now my sister has been killed by a warring *zamindar* faction. I don't want this way of life. That's why I am going to Benares."

"But you are a young man, barely into your twenties," the women objected. "You are not at the age to become an ascetic. You should come with us."

Perhaps he could begin a new life without taking the vows of asceticism, Ram Chandra thought. He joined the two women as they traveled to the city of Jessore. From there he made his way to Dhaka where he found work, married again, and began a family. Eventually he acquired property, but, still attracted to asceticism, he gave away most of the land, saying, "We don't want it; what we have is sufficient for us."

Malay paused, as though to let the story sink into my western mind, unaccustomed to *zamindars* and ascetics and pilgrimages to holy cities. Then he repeated his thesis. "This tradition of forsaking properties has been going on since then," he said. "Bela fits that tradition. She has very little attachment to things that other people value greatly."

Bela's father Mukunda Chandra Banerjee also had been influenced by Ram Chandra. Although, like his ancestors, Mukunda was a *zamindar*, he was also a schoolmaster who tried to improve the quality of education in the area where he lived. In Mukunda's time, Malay told me, the British had only one purpose in their administration of land owned by the *zamindars*: to collect taxes on the property. Social services, if there were any, were the responsibilities of the *zamindars*.

In the region where Bela's father owned property, the most influential *zamindar* was a woman who, like Mukunda, was concerned for the welfare of the people. The lady *zamindar*, as she was called, had started several schools in her *zamindari*. Mukunda Banerjee was convinced that if the Indian people were to advance under British rule, they must have opportunity to learn English. With this concern he went to the lady *zamindar*, suggesting that students should have the option of receiving an English education instead of only attending vernacular schools. The lady *zamindar* respected Mukunda Banerjee's ideas; following his suggestion, she started an English-medium high school in the small town of Shantash and asked him to be the headmaster. Mukunda moved into the hostel to live with the students, returning to his family in his home village of Butani only for holidays.

Satish Banerjee, Mukunda's oldest son, studied in his father's school until he went to the university in Calcutta. Satish shared his father's concern for the advancement of his people. One way in which he expressed his concern was to participate in the national movement, which at that time shortly after the turn of the century opposed the British division of Bengal. Much of northeastern India was a part of Bengal, but the British had divided the state into two parts, with East Bengal and Assam forming one province and West Bengal, Bihar and Orissa combined into another. Satish was one of many young men who visited villages and towns in several districts in an attempt to organize people against the division. Ultimately the two parts of Bengal were reunited (only to be divided again with independence); however, in the new arrangements the states of Assam, Bihar, and Orissa were separated from Bengal.

Satish, like his forebears, felt little attachment to material possessions. On a trip to Butani during the time he was responsible for his father's property, for example, Satish noted the poverty of the tenant farmers and gave them the fisheries project that belonged to the *zamindari*. Except for his share of the inheritance of his father's land which he and his brothers sold, Satish never owned property.

Bela has no memories of the village of Butani where she lived as a small child. For Bela those years exist only in the stories her mother told her, mostly after she was grown. Once she came to make her home with Satish, Bela never went back. Unconsciously, however, Bela's early life in Butani must have had a lasting influence on her. When her nephew Samiran told me about Butani, I sensed a connection between Bela's village origin and her identification with villagers among whom she has worked as a nurse.

Like Malay, Samiran is a story-teller. "I have been to that village, to the house where she was born," he began. I sat back, imagining the experience that Samiran was obviously reliving as he talked. "From Calcutta you start out by train," he said. "It's a whole night of train travel. In the morning—early morning—you come to a port, Aricha."

Samiran scarcely paused as he shifted the setting of the story. "You go in a boat some distance farther, traveling from midnight to six a.m., before you continue the journey on land. Then you go by what is called *ekka*," Samiran said, giving the Bengali name to the one-horse cart and driver whose services were required to travel from the shore to the village. Samiran remembered the condition of the road. "A very difficult road. Muddy sometimes."

He described the village of Butani and the Banerjee home where Bela had been born. "The village is full of fruit trees—mangoes and leechies, various other fruits. These trees belong to the people who live there. You go along a single-lane road, just one person's width. And then you come to a small house, a shrine, where my grandmother used to worship."

Samiran told me about the mud houses in the compound, surrounded by bamboo fencing. "Quite nice," he said. "Neat and clean. On one side my aunts used to live, and my grandmother. On the other side were oxen and storerooms. Another part was a large food storage place for *muri*, rice, and *dhal*. In a big room nearby, my uncle lived with his family.

"I could see that they had had quite a good life at one time," Samiran said. He told about seeing silver bowls and stone plates and bronze utensils in his grandmother's home, beautiful items that she eventually gave to relatives in the compound.

According to Samiran, Bela's mother received income from coconut and mango trees and paddy fields. However, because the man in charge of her land was a poor manager, she got very little.

When Samiran visited Bela's mother in the village, she showed him a long veranda where she used to serve big feasts when her husband was still living. "Relatives would come and sit down and say, 'let us have a good feast.' And then she would cook—all things, whatever they wanted. She showed me the banana trees where they used to cut the leaves for the plates."

Samiran went on, telling the outcome of his step grandmother's generosity. "She thought that whenever her money would run short, they would give her money or bring her food, and she could carry on like that. But they didn't. After the money was gone, they disappeared. When nothing was left, she was in great difficulty."

When she went to live with Satish, Bela's mother still owned the land and received some income from the crops after every harvest. Later Bela's brother and half brothers sold the land. By then all three of them lived in Calcutta. When Bela's uncle in the village also moved to Calcutta with his family some years later, the Banerjee family ties to the village of Butani were completely cut.

Bela's brother Monesh became a dentist, married, and had one child, a boy, who grew up to become a lawyer in Delhi. When Chandron, his son, was still a baby, Monesh suddenly disappeared. Satish heard from Monesh once after he left his home; then he was in Bombay. Bela was in England at the time, but when she returned and tried to locate Monesh, she found no trace of him anywhere. Monesh had vanished during a period of Hindu-Moslem riots at the time of partition in the mid-1940s, and the family speculated that he had been killed in the riots.

Soon after Monesh's disappearance, his wife Indira took Chandron and moved to her parents' home near Delhi. Bela and Indira kept in touch. As soon as Bela had enough income, she sent 50 *rupees* a month to Indira for Chandron's education, a practice she continued until he graduated from the university and started practicing law. Every year for the gift-giving holiday of the *Durga Puja*, Monesh's wife sends a new *sari* to Bela. When Bela occasionally goes to Delhi, she stays with Indira. At Indira's home Bela also keeps a trunk of letters and a few other possessions that she has not carried with her when she has moved.

Bela's family ties to her sister Sushama and to Satish's children are strong. Whenever possible, she visits in their homes when she travels to West Bengal. Her Banerjee heritage is important to her. Other Banerjee family members who share that heritage say that it is Bela more than any of them who has continued the tradition of simplicity that their ancestor Ram Chandra Banerjee began.

Along with choosing a simple way of life, Bela has enlarged her philosophy to include all people in her sense of family. Her nephew Samiran summarized it this way: "She went to the Moslem area in the worst slum of Calcutta; she went to Kerala where a different people spoke another language; she went to Orissa where again the people were different—everywhere she found one family. She went to England; she went to America—all that she met are members of that one family. This oneness guides her life."

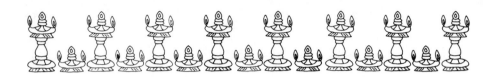

4
CHILDHOOD MEMORIES

Bela and her niece Jutika reminisced about their childhood, as we visited over tea and sweets at Jutika's home in the south part of Calcutta. Jutika named all the places the Banerjees had lived after Bela's family came to stay with them. Although they considered Calcutta to be their permanent home, the Banerjees frequently moved for short periods of time to a more healthful environment in Bihar. Bela and Jutika tried to remember how many months or years they had remained in each location.

"So many places we lived. So many times we moved," Bela said. She described how she had packed things into trunks. "It was mostly bedding and clothing. We didn't have much furniture, and we purchased wooden cots when we got there. But we took everything from the house with every move. And we loaded all the things onto the third class train along with our big load of people," she said.

When they thought about their home on Raja Dinendra Street in Calcutta, the first memory that came to Jutika and Bela was the birth of Jutika's youngest sister Pushbanjali on the last day of 1927. Together they told me the story.

When the doctor had arrived in the evening, all the children were sent away from the room where the delivery was to take place. Although Bela and her nieces were excited by the prospect of the new baby's arrival, they were also staying awake because it was New Year's Eve. At midnight a neighborhood band began to play, welcoming the new year. Shortly afterwards, someone reported to the waiting youngsters that a baby girl had been born just before the new year arrived.

To Bela it was as if the New Year's Eve band was announcing the birth. In her imagination, a special relationship with her youngest niece had already begun, even before it was daylight and her mother took her to Kripa's room to see the new baby.

At first Bela was not allowed to hold Pushbanjali, because Kripa was concerned about infections being spread to the new baby through contact with other children. "My sister and my mother took care of her," Bela remembered, "but they said I wasn't big enough."

When Pushbanjali was about three months old, the day finally arrived that Bela could help take care of her. "I started by giving her a bath," Bela remembered. "I put soap on her and washed her. She was such a beautiful child, really," Bela went on. "I used to play with her, and I was so fond of her. I never felt bad about cleaning her." When Pushbanjali was weaned, Bela eagerly took on the duties of feeding her.

After traveling a morning's journey from Calcutta to Pushbanjali's home in Kharagpur, I heard about Pushbanjali's first memory of Bela. "We were living in Santal Pagana in Bihar," Pushbanjali said. "I was crying and making quite a fuss about a boil I had on my forehead. I was suffering very badly, and nobody could do anything about it. But I loved my aunt dearly, and when she said, 'If I pick you up, will you stop wailing?' I quit crying. I remember we were standing near a well in the courtyard of our home, and she held me and comforted me."

Without a pause Pushbanjali continued, speaking of the qualities Bela manifested in her relationships with family members. "She was so loving and soft-hearted, always trying to do things for others. And she always had a smile," Pushbanjali said.

When Bela and her niece Shefalika visited with me in Shefalika's second story flat in a large apartment house in north Calcutta, the memories they recounted were about marriage, specifically the Indian custom of arranged marriage and how it related to their lives.

When Bela and Shefalika became teenagers, Satish, at his wife's suggestion, began to look for husbands for both girls at the same time. Bela knew, however, that their qualifications were not equal. Although she had a pleasant nature, Bela was exceedingly thin. She had sharp features and slightly protruding teeth. She was sure that her appearance, coupled with her poverty and lack of education, stood in the way of a good match. "No dowry. Ugly-looking. No money. No education." She listed her faults as she told me about her brother's search. "Nobody would want to marry me, that I knew," she said.

Shefalika had a different point of view about Bela's prospects. "I thought that Bela would get married because of her training in the household management and work," she said.

As it turned out, neither of the two married. Shefalika remained single because her father could not find a young man that he considered suitable for her to marry. She became a teacher.

For Bela, Satish had set different standards. He came to her one day and said, "I have found someone you can marry."

"By then I had the feeling that if I got married I would just make another poor family with too many children, and I didn't want to do it," Bela said to me. "I would like to have had my own babies—I am very fond of children, you know—but I saw some marriages that were not really very happy. And so I said, 'No, I'm not going to get married.'"

Bela decided she would prefer to continue to do housework in exchange for a place in Satish's home. "I thought that is what I would do the rest of my life, and I was quite happy," she told me.

More than the Brahman caste to which Bela belonged by birth, the Brahmo Samaj faith that Satish practiced was in keeping with the pattern of life that Bela chose for herself. "I was very attached to my oldest brother," Bela told me, explaining that she was influenced by Satish's values. "He was like a father to me. I held him in great respect."

Bela's youngest niece recognized that her father had played a great role in Bela's life. "The dedication to helping others with his own earnings that I saw in my father I also see in my aunt," Pushbanjali told me.

"She is a product of the main Brahmo spirit," added Pushbanjali's husband Dipankar Niyogin, attributing Satish's religious values to Bela.

Each of Bela's nieces and nephews whom I met listed the major tenets of the Brahmo Samaj, using the traditional wording of their statement of faith. "Do good to others is the Brahmo ideal. We believe in the brotherhood of man and the fatherhood of God. Because that is so, there cannot be any caste system or hierarchy in society or economic class. We do not believe in superstition or the worship of idols, but think that we should always exercise rationality. Education and culture and cultivation of your faculties are important. Work is worship."

Shefalika told me, "Brahmo Samaj is something you join. There is a ceremony for new members and they make a promise, a vow.

Children of Brahmo Samaj members do not have to make vows in order to be members."

I asked Bela if she had joined. "No, I didn't join, but I was brought up with it. My mind was like that," she said. "I used to go to their meetings."

Bela explained the Brahmo Samaj by saying they were much like the Quakers with whom she worked for many years after she left Satish's home. "That is why I like the Quakers so much, because I was brought up in a Quaker"—she stopped to correct herself—"Brahmo Samaj family."

Bela's Brahmo Samaj background prepared her not only for her ties to Quaker development work, but also for her later involvement in Gandhian social service projects. With independence from Great Britain in 1947, many of the social concerns of both the Brahmo Samaj and the Gandhian movements were written into the Indian constitution. However, it is only as individuals such as Bela Banerjee have implemented those concerns that the daily lives of the Indian people have been affected.

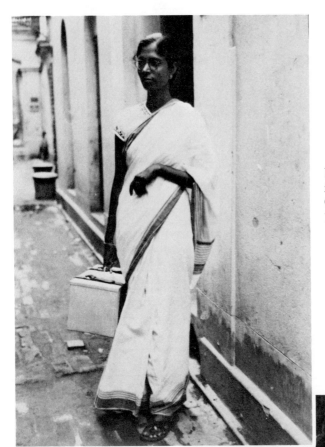

Bela carrying her midwifery kit to a delivery in a Calcutta home, mid-1940s.

The Calcutta neighborhood where Bela and Joan Court worked with the Friends Service Unit, 1946.

PART TWO:

CALCUTTA: WORK AMONG THE POOR

"Who among you will take up the duty of feeding the hungry?" Lord Buddha asked his followers when famine raged at Shravasti.

Ratnakar, the banker, hung his head and said, "Much more is needed than all my wealth to feed the hungry."

Jaysen, the chief of the King's army, said, "I would gladly give my life's blood, but there is not enough food in my house."

Dharmapal, who owned broad acres of land, said with a sigh, "The drought demon has sucked my fields dry. I know not how to pay King's dues."

Then rose Supriya, the mendicant's daughter.

She bowed to all and meekly said, "I will feed the hungry."

"How!" they cried in surprise. "How can you hope to fulfill that vow?"

"I am the poorest of you all," said Supriya, "that is my strength. I have my coffer and my store at each of your houses."

—Rabindranath Tagore
"Fruit-Gathering XXXI"

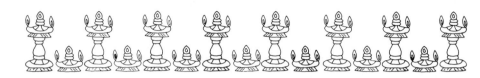

5

THE BENGAL SOCIAL SERVICE LEAGUE

The car in which Bela Banerjee and I were riding turned from the main thoroughfare near Calcutta's Sealdah Railroad Station into the Raja-bazaar area of the city. Immediately the neighborhood looked different. The road was narrower. Cattle wandered about. A bullock cart was parked next to the sidewalk. Except that the large two-story houses were like those in other parts of the city, it appeared as though a Bengali village had been left in place when the city pushed out its boundaries. "When I lived here, there were mud huts with thatched roofs," Bela said. "It was almost at the very edge of Calcutta then," she added.

We stopped beside the Bengal Social Service League, a large, yellow brick building on Raja Dinendra Street, the location of Bela's first job outside Satish's home. As Bela and I got out of the car, we were surrounded by a crowd of laughing, shouting children who had seen the camera around my neck and wanted to have their pictures taken.

Four women in cotton *saris* looked out from their doorways at the commotion. They recognized Bela and came running to greet her. She tried to introduce the women to me, but the press of noisy children prevented easy conversation. I decided to take a picture of Bela with her friends and moved back a few feet to focus my camera. That was a mistake. Immediately the children filled every inch of space. They shouted, jostled one another, and waved their hands in front of the camera.

Bela suggested that we go inside the building to visit. We made our way to the corner entrance of the Bengal Social Service League, but a dozen children reached the door before us and pushed into the building. Just as we got inside, two men with frightened eyes snapped shut a heavy iron gate that cut off the entrance-way from the lobby. Bela spoke to them through the grille. "I used to work here many years ago, and we have come back to visit," she said.

"You could be starting a riot," one of the men responded. "There is much unrest in this area." He turned to me. "Take your camera and get back into your car at once," he said.

It looked to me like the normal reaction of children who seldom see outsiders, but I obeyed the order. The children followed me to the street, their antics still begging to be photographed.

Bela was not willing to leave her friends until she at least asked how many grandchildren they had and what had happened to their children whom she had known as toddlers. They stood on the sidewalk, talking.

Finally Bela came to the car, her smile and her eyes beaming in her elation over having seen the four women. "When I first knew those women, they were in *purdah*," she said, reflecting on their freedom now to come out into the street unaccompanied, their faces uncovered.

"How did you recognize them?" I asked. If they had been secluded behind a *burkha*, the head to foot covering of Moslem women in *purdah*, I wondered how she would have known what they looked like.

"I used to visit them in their homes. And when they came to the Social Service League, I took them to the roof top where no one would see them, so they could take off their *burkhas* and get sunlight. Before that, they all had Vitamin D deficiencies," she said.

Bela's work at the Bengal Social Service League began in June 1935, after she had lived in Satish's home for about ten years. By then Sushama had married and Monesh had settled into his school routine. Bela had taken over most of the household responsibilities; her mother had returned to their village home, hoping that her health might be better there than in Calcutta. For a year or more Satish sent five *rupees* a month to Bela's mother in the village (Rs.5 = U.S.$1.65 then). But, because his income did not provide for his large family as well as it had when he was younger, Satish decided that he could no longer afford to send money to his stepmother every month.

"I wanted very much to look after my mother," Bela told me. "I thought she needed some help and I knew it was difficult for my brother to give help, so I decided I would try to find a way to go out and earn some money."

While Bela was wondering what kind of job she could do and how she would go about finding a place to work for pay, Jhunu Bhose, the daughter of Kripa's sister Balukana, came to see her. Whenever Jhunu had visited the Banerjee home, she had noticed how hard Bela worked, whether in the routine care of the household or in the preparation of the feasts that the Banerjees served at celebrations. Learning that Bela was looking for a job in order to earn some money, Jhunu was ready with a suggestion. "They want to hire a matron to look after the ladies' hostel at the Bengal Social Service League," she told Bela. "They will pay ten *rupees*."

"I got so excited," Bela told me, laughing as she thought about it. "Ten *rupees*! I wanted to earn five *rupees* a month to send my mother, but I got ten *rupees*. Pocket money. And they would give me my food, too. And a room. I was very, very happy."

Jhunu's parents, Balukana and Nishisantababu Bhose, both worked at the Bengal Social Service League, a Brahmo Samaj project in a Moslem slum area in the northern part of Calcutta. Dr. Dijendranath Moitra, who was in charge of the institution, had started the project to put into practice the Brahmo Samaj belief in the interrelatedness of all people.

Balukana helped Bela to apply for the job, writing a recommendation for her to Dr. Moitra. "She wrote that I was very good as a housekeeper because I had looked after my brother's big house for his large family," Bela recalled. "But she added four years onto the age that we guessed I was at the time, because she thought I was not old enough for the job."

Bela's job as matron of the hostel was to manage the household accounts and plan the meals for the 25 to 30 young women who lived there.

Sabitri-devi was one of the young women staying at the hostel when Bela became the matron. All of the other women were students at the nearby Women's Training College for Teachers, but Sabitri was still studying in high school. Drawn together because they were younger than the other women, Bela's closeness with Sabitri was established on a more deeply shared experience than their age: both girls had encountered unusual hardships in their lives.

Daughter of a physician who was also a village *zamindar*, Sabitri had never experienced the deprivation and hard work that had been a part of Bela's life, but she had suffered in a different way. In the first place, Sabitri was a child widow. Within a year after her marriage at 13, her husband had died. Moreover, before she was 15, she had spent three months in jail for delivering a speech against the British at a rally for national independence. By the time she met Bela, Sabitri's participation in the independence movement had resulted in three prison sentences.

Bela took me to visit Sabitri in her North Calcutta home. "I am a political sufferer," Sabitri told me in English and then switched to Bengali. "Being among the poor people, just witnessing their critical conditions affected me deeply. I was inspired to help those people who were suffering. Whenever I found someone who was suffering, I took it to be my responsibility to help that person."

"So that's why your friendship with Bela is so close?" I asked.

She spoke again in English. "I love her very much."

Sabitri said that when Bela came to the hostel at the Bengal Social Service League, she brought with her a torn sheet and two torn *saris*. "I took them and threw them away and shared my own with her," she said.

Bela laughed, recalling the incident, but putting down its significance. "I'm still like that," she said. "I still use my *saris* and sheets when they are torn."

Having entered the conversation, Bela began telling other examples of Sabitri's concern for her. "She used to worry about me— whether I was eating or not, for example. You know, sometimes I used to feel that I was too poor and was giving people a lot of trouble, and so I didn't tell people that I hadn't eaten. But Sabitri-devi would find out, and she used to say, 'Whether you have eaten or not you have to eat with me before you can go out.'"

From the beginning Sabitri was protective of Bela. If any one at the hostel criticized her cooking, Bela would start to cry. Sabitri would defend her, demanding angrily, "Why are you talking to her like that?"

Bela made friends quickly with the women at the hostel, and in the evenings when they studied, she would join them, eager to absorb new knowledge. She often borrowed books from Sisir Kana-devi, a woman who had been headmistress of a middle school. Sisir Kana was married and had a baby; sometimes she took Bela home with her on holidays. Occasionally they went to a cinema or to the Botanical Gardens on the outskirts of Calcutta.

During the evenings at the hostel, Bela most often studied with Sabitri. "English. Bengali. Math. History. Whatever she was studying, I would read." Bela said.

Sabitri sometimes made tea to drink to help her stay awake while she studied. Bela had often served tea to others, but she had seldom been offered tea; at first she protested when Sabitri brought her a cup to drink. "If you make me have the habit to drink tea, who will give me tea when I have no money and have to buy it?"

"That's all right," Sabitri had retorted. "Whenever you need money for tea, I will always give it."

"Then I can drink tea with you now," Bela had answered with a laugh.

The joke between them had continued through the years. When Bela went to Sabitri's house a few days before I arrived, she asked Sabitri if she remembered the promise to give her money for tea when she needed it. Sabitri had said, "Has it happened like that, that you cannot have a cup of tea? Have you a problem in getting the money for a cup of tea?"

"No."

"Then when you have that condition that you have no money for a cup of tea—when you have that problem—you come, and I will give the money to you. Certainly I will give it to you."

Bela and I had tea, and later a meal, in Sabitri's home where she lives with her 90-year-old widowed brother Sri Sinha and two generations of his descendants. A friendly family from the Bania caste who traditionally were businessmen and money lenders, the Sinhas welcomed Bela and me into their home. It was the same house where, in years past, Bela had visited and had helped Sabitri to take care of Sabitri's invalid stepmother.

I noticed that the Sinhas greeted Bela as if she were a daughter in the family. Even the youngest grandson called her *chhordi*, which means "little sister," an affectionate name he had picked up from his parents, grandfather, and great-aunt Sabitri.

In the small front room where we sat to visit at the Sinha home, a copper plaque hung on the wall—a tribute to Sabitri Das's role as a freedom fighter. In 1972, on the 25th anniversary of India's independence from England, Sabitri was among the hundreds of survivors of the independence movement who were honored with the citation plaque and a monthly pension for the rest of their lives.

While she was working at the Bengal Social Service League, Bela became friends with Sati, a young woman who came frequently to visit Lela, the headmistress in a school that the league had organized for neighborhood children. After Sati married Bhupen Ghose, Bela often visited them when she went to see Satish's family, whose home was nearby. It was with Sati and Bhupen and their son's family that Bela and I stayed for several days when we were in Calcutta as we traveled together in 1982. Theirs was another of the homes where Bela was considered to be a member of the family. "I know I could come to them at any time of the day or night," Bela said of her years of friendship with the Ghoses.

Even though she earned very little, Bela's work at the Bengal Social Service League provided her—for the first time in her life—with money to spend as she chose. Each month she sent five *rupees* to her mother in the village. From the five *rupees* that remained, she saved nearly a rupee a month.

By the end of the first six months she had saved five rupees, enough to buy Pushbanjali, her favorite niece, a bottle of Evening in Paris cologne for her birthday.

In the way she chose to spend her earnings in her first job at the Bengal Social Service League, Bela began a practice that she has followed ever since. Except for meeting her own barest needs, she has always used her money for others. Through the years, most members of her family and many of her friends were helped by her generosity.

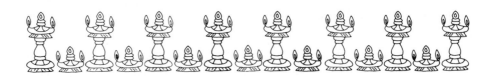

6
CLINIC WORK WITH LIES GOMPERTZ

A conversation about Bela Banerjee's work at the Bengal Social Service League, whether with her or anyone who knew her there, does not go far before the importance of Lies Gompertz in Bela's life is made clear. It was with Lies that Bela began health work among poor women and children of India.

Lies, a nurse, was a Jewish refugee who came to India during the mid-thirties to escape the repression that was developing in Hitler's Germany.

She was hired by Dr. Dijendranath Moitra to broaden the work of the Bengal Social Service League by providing health care services for children of the Rajabazaar neighborhood. At first her main activity was to distribute milk and provide hygienic care in a program funded by the Calcutta Corporation, the municipal social service agency. After about a year she expanded her work to include a clinic for mothers and babies.

Dr. Moitra asked Bela to assist Lies in addition to her work at the hostel. When the Teachers Training College, where most of the hostel residents were studying, was shut down because of bombings during the Second World War, Dr. Moitra closed the hostel and Bela worked with Lies full time.

All of Bela's friends whom I met in Calcutta talked about Lies Gompertz. Sabitri began her reminiscences by telling about her initial memory of Lies. "When Lies first came, she worried about bugs," Sabitri said. "She started cleaning everything up because of the bugs. She thought everything was a bug." Sabitri laughed at her own exaggeration.

Bela joined in the laughter and then changed the subject. "Lies and I used to work together, you know. And because I couldn't speak English, whenever she was doing anything, I used to go and just do the same as she was doing."

Sabitri seemed to catch the focus of Bela's thought, and she added. "Lies was a help to Bela and loved her so much."

Not all of Bela's friends remembered Lies in the same generous light. One of her acquaintances told me that Lies controlled Bela unnecessarily. "She thought that if any good was to be done to Bela it must be done through her—Lies; nobody else could do that," he complained.

"She was protective of me," Bela suggested.

"Not protecting her. Possessing her," he retorted.

I pressed for details. From the conversation that ensued, I concluded that the man, a teen-age college student at the time he first knew Bela, liked to visit her in the evenings because she would cook snacks that he enjoyed eating; when he tried to expand his visits by coming in the afternoon as well, Lies intervened, saying that Bela needed to rest after the strenuous work of the morning.

Bela laughed. "Lies used to say, 'Now she will put her legs up and her head down,' and then she would put a pillow under my feet and say, 'you should rest.'"

"As you did with me today," I said, remembering how, that afternoon, insisting that I rest, Bela had swept my feet off the floor and onto the cot where I was sitting.

Bela nodded. "Lies is the one who taught me all these things. What she has taught me I have kept all my life. I don't need to have learned anything more. She was really so good to me." Bela seemed intent on offsetting criticism of Lies with heightened praise. "Lies was the most important influence of my life," Bela told me on another occasion. "She took so much interest and wanted to help me all the way. In everything she was so sincere. She really loved people. In every way she taught me."

Bela went on to tell how she and Lies developed a pattern of working together. The first work that they did was to organize a maternal and child health center at the Social Service League. Because Bela understood very little English and Lies did not know Bengali, Bela learned what to do by watching Lies the first day.

On the second day, before Lies was awake, Bela went to the room where food was to be distributed and did the things she had seen Lies do the day before. By the time Lies arrived the second morning, Bela had boiled milk for the children and was cooking porridge and semolina for the mothers and babies to eat. She had gotten out the aluminum jugs in which the milk would be distributed to the families of the neighborhood.

When Lies arrived that morning and saw what Bela had done, she said, "Bela, you are really wonderful." Bela smiled and used her limited English vocabulary to say, "Thank you, Lies." Gradually as they worked together, Bela learned more English and a few words of German, Lies's native tongue; Lies also learned some Bengali from Bela. The *bustee* residents who came to the clinic spoke a dialect of Hindi rather than Bengali. Along with trying to learn enough English to communicate with Lies, Bela visited the mothers in their homes so that she could learn the local dialect.

In late afternoons and early evenings, she and Lies visited homes of the women who were receiving prenatal or postnatal care. Lies gave follow-up treatment to patients who had been at the clinic and Bela practiced her Hindi by talking to the women and their children.

The first time Lies asked Bela to treat a patient without her help turned out to be a traumatic experience for Bela even before she went to the patient's home. Bela and Lies had gone to the rooftop so that Lies could point out the house that Bela was to visit.

Lies began to describe the woman's condition. "Lies was explaining about a breast abscess that she had tried to drain in the morning, but couldn't, and she was telling me how to do it," Bela said. Lies' graphic description of the woman's condition and the treatment she wanted Bela to administer was overwhelming for Bela, who had up to then given only sympathy to the patients. "I fainted," she said, continuing the story. "My mother was there with us, and she was terribly frightened. She started crying and saying that I was dead. But Lies carried me to her room, and I was all right in a few minutes. I didn't go to that house that day, but I went later."

Each day except Sunday 40 or 50 children from the neighborhood came to the big lecture hall on the ground floor of the Social Service League. Lies and Bela bathed the children at a water tap in a corner of the room near a drain in the cement floor. They shampooed and combed the children's hair and applied the insecticide gamaxene to the children's scalps, attempting to get rid of the lice that infested most of the children. After the baths were finished, each child drank a cup of milk and then sat on the floor to draw or write on a slate that Bela and Lies provided.

While the children were downstairs in the big hall, Bela took some of their mothers to the rooftop of the four-story building, so that they could sit in the sun and take off their *burkhas*. The mothers took their small babies along, and Bela rubbed the babies' bodies all over with cod-liver oil.

As the clinic developed, Bela assisted Lies in offering prenatal care, encouraging pregnant women to call a Calcutta Corporation midwife for their deliveries or to go to the hospital if complications were likely. After the babies were born, Lies and Bela provided postnatal care, largely through a program of improved nutrition. To mothers of malnourished babies, they gave extra calcium. For all the nursing mothers, they made a porridge of cream of wheat, called *sujee*. They fed a similar porridge, thinned with milk, to the babies who were over three months in age, adding spinach, carrots, and potatoes to the porridge for older infants.

Besides distributing food at the daily maternal and child health clinic, Bela and Lies weighed the babies and talked to the pregnant women about their diets and the importance of cleanliness at childbirth.

The clinic was held near the lecture hall at the Social Service League in four small rooms that were converted to an examining room, a kitchen, a waiting room, and a room for medicine cupboards.

Some of Bela's nieces and nephews visited her occasionally at the Bengal Social Service League. Pushbanjali had just started to school at the time that Bela went to the Bengal Social Service League to work—often she spent time with Bela when she was not in school. "I was very fond of her, and I used to go and stay with her and follow her around,' Pushbanjali told me. "I remember the slum people from Rajabazaar coming to the Social Service League to get milk."

Bela's nephew Samiran Banerjee had thought he might be interested in working with slum residents when he finished his education, so after Bela started to work at the Bengal Social Service League, he visited her to see what it would be like. "I found my aunt sitting there with dirty-clothed children—very dirty—and they all cuddled up to her. And their parents, chewing *pan* (a betel nut concoction) and spitting the red juice anywhere—I couldn't stand it; after a few minutes I felt almost suffocated. But she was just smiling and writing down their answers when she asked them why they had come to the clinic. And if one of the children had an accident she would say, 'Oh, dear, that's all right. Come.' And she would take him to the toilet and clean him up. I was quite amazed to see what patience and tolerance she had."

When India entered World War II through England's declaration of war against Germany in September 1939, life changed at the Social Service League, as it did everywhere in Calcutta and in the country as a whole. At the League the most direct changes were related to the fact that the nearby schools where hostel residents had attended were closed because of occasional bombing. Even when the schools were open, there was a shortage of teachers. Dr. Moitra decided to close the hostel and use its facilities for other work.

Because Lies was a German citizen, twice she was interned in a detention center in Darjeeling. One internment lasted about a month and the other about three months. Both times Dr. Moitra intervened, using his influence with the British authorities to obtain her release.

While Lies was confined in the detention camp, she and Bela exchanged letters. Bela had difficulty reading Lies's letters, which were written in English, so she took them to her friend Sati Ghose, whose husband Bhupen translated for her. Bhupen teased Bela about it afterwards, telling me that when Bela got a letter from Lies she would bring it to him and say, "Read it to me, and after reading, answer also that letter." Actually, to answer Lies' letters, Bela wrote what she wanted to say in Bengali for Bhupen to translate into English. Then, using pen and ink, Bela copied what Bhupen had written.

Bela's work during Lies's internment was expanded to include the duties in which she previously had only assisted. At another time, when Lies required surgery and a long period of recuperation outside Calcutta, Bela also took charge of the clinic, as well as the orphanage that had begun by then.

The work with orphans had been started in 1942, after a crop failure in Bengal. The crop failure, added to the fact that government food reserves had been used for the army during the war mobilization, resulted in a severe famine throughout the state. The famine lasted for about three years. All over Calcutta, people who could afford to cook rice and *dhal* in their homes took food to soup kitchens set up by the government to feed the thousands of people who streamed into the city from the barren countryside.

Bela's niece Pushbanjali described the effects of the famine as she remembered it: "It was a terrible thing. People went from door to door asking for—not rice, even—but just a little rice water." Hundreds of people died of starvation, and many children were orphaned.

Dr. Moitra opened the Social Service League to care for 15 orphans. The children stayed in the second story rooms that previously had been the ladies' hostel. Six older girls came to Bengal Social Service League to help take care of the children. Lies and Bela organized a training program for the girls, some of whom had come from within the local neighborhood. The Indian Red Cross and the

Save the Children Fund cooperated with the Bengal Social Service League to finance the training program and the orphanage.

Lies and Bela's work became well known around Calcutta. The Government Welfare Center sent its workers to the Bengal Social Service League on field trips to see an example of a well-run center, pointing out how the orphanage and the training of workers were intermeshed with the clinic work among the neighborhood residents in a successful blend of health care.

At the Bengal Social Service League, while working with Lies, Bela began to focus on the methods of development that turned out to be integral to her work when she became a nurse in charge of health programs in village development projects. This was also the first of several projects where Bela helped to train health workers.

Three characteristics of Bela's working style at the Bengal Social Service League have continued throughout her working years. Her first step in each new location has been to become well acquainted with the local people by visiting their homes and learning their language. A second major focus of her approach has been to teach health concepts to families by working with their children. The third unique feature of her style of working has been to train local girls to implement the health program.

During the time she worked at the Bengal Social Service League, Bela began to develop her philosophy of working with people to help their own neighbors live more healthful lives. Bela believes that people do most things by habit, so she thinks it is important to focus on improved health and hygiene standards at an early age.

"Did you get that idea from Lies?" I asked.

"No, I don't think Lies had that idea. She showed me how to do the work, but it was my own idea—the importance of starting with children in forming habits. And still I have the feeling that that's the way. I'm still working that way.

"The idea of going to visit people in their homes and learning how to talk to them, how to give advice—those things I learned from Lies. And the clinic work."

Lies and Bela had not worked together long when Bela's mother returned to Calcutta from her village home, sharing Bela's room at the Social Service League. At first Bela's mother had difficulty adjusting to life at the Bengal Social Service League. Her traditional Brahman standards were an obstacle in relating to the orphan children. "Why did you bring me here among these untouchables?" she would complain to Bela. Gradually, as the children continued their practice of coming to see Bela in her room and included her mother in their affection, calling her "grandmother," Bela's mother softened her attitude and eventually she became fond of the children. "She started to like them, then to love them," Bela said. She began to teach the older girls how to embroider and to sew, and she took pleasure in combing the younger children's hair.

When Bela began to work with Lies, her salary was raised, first to 15 *rupees* and then to 25 *rupees*. When the orphanage and training program were started, the Red Cross began to underwrite the cost of the program, and for the first time Bela received something more than pocket money—wages of 150 *rupees* every month. Immediately she started sending 50 *rupees* a month to Satish for Pushbanjali's education. Frequently she sent gifts of up to ten *rupees* at a time to her sister's small children, giving them an opportunity to have their own spending money—an experience that she and her sister had never had when they were children.

Sometimes when Bela ran out of money she pawned her gold necklace and two gold bangles, taking them to a jeweler near the Bengal Social Service League. The jeweler, one of Bela's friends in the neighborhood, had originally made the jewelry from a gold coin that Bela's mother had saved for her.

In addition to the Moslem slum neighbors, other families lived in the area near the Bengal Social Service League. Many of them were members of the Brahmo Samaj who had moved to the neighborhood to establish other service agencies to help the poor. Adjoining the Bengal Social Service League was an adult education and literacy center that included a multi-purpose school for teaching weaving and other handicrafts. Gnananjon Niyogin, who ran the institution, lived with his family on the top floor of the building.

Bela became good friends with Roma, the Niyogin daughter who was about her age. The two young women enjoyed going for walks together in a nearby Ladies' Park. Sometimes Roma's mother invited Bela to eat with the family. Dipankar, Roma's little brother, became a favorite friend of Bela's. Lonely because he had few playmates nearby, Dipankar appreciated the attention. When he was about ten years old, his room was on the third floor terrace which overlooked the flat rooftop of the Bengal Social Service League. Sometimes when Bela was on the rooftop they would visit. At least once a week Bela's mother invited Dipankar to their room to eat something that she had cooked, "Lovely dishes," he said, describing to me the Bengali sweets Bela's mother shared with him when he was a little boy.

While Bela was at the Bengal Social Service League she needed to get glasses, but she did not know where to go. A young woman who lived at the hostel took her to Abdullah Mallik, a Moslem doctor who later (following partition) became a member of the Pakistani government. Dr. Mallik was especially kind to Bela, giving her the glasses at cost. When Bela's mother needed medical care, Bela sought Dr. Mallik's advice. He referred her to another doctor, asking him not to take any money from Bela because she was working to help the poor. "He was very kind to me all the time," Bela said.

Dr. Mallik's home was near his office. Sometimes Bela visited Mrs. Mallik, who was from Austria, and their two children. At the time, Dr. Mallik's daughter was studying at the Brahmo Samaj Girls' School in Calcutta. Knowing that Bela came from a Brahmo Samaj family and lived very simply, he sometimes likened his daughter to her. Calling Bela his sister, he would say to her, "My daughter is just like her aunt. She doesn't care for fancy clothes or anything. She lives simply, like you."

———————————

A neighborhood jeweler, a little boy next door, a Moslem doctor: Bela became friends with the people she met in the ordinary experiences of her day-to-day work, and in their homes she was treated as a family member.

At the Bengal Social Service League, Bela began to feel as much at home as she had when she lived with Satish's family, and she had the same attitude toward her work as when she had managed Satish's household. "I thought that is what I would always do, and I was quite content," she said.

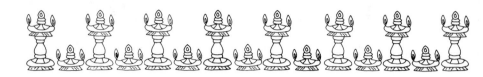

7
MIDWIFERY TRAINING

Bela had been Lies Gompertz's assistant for several years, when Lies decided Bela should take a midwifery course at the Lady Dufferin Victoria Memorial Hospital in Calcutta. Not deterred by the fact that Bela had never been to school, Lies set about to get the requirement of high school graduation waived for the English-medium midwifery course.

She contacted two people who wrote statements of recommendation for Bela. Sisir Kana-devi, who had helped Bela with her informal studies at the Bengal Social Service League hostel, stated that Bela had the equivalent of a high school education. An English Red Cross doctor who brought supplies each week to the Bengal Social Service League clinic described his observation of Bela's work and requested that the graduation requirement be waived because of her experience. Lies took the two documents to Dr. Neal, Superintendent of Lady Dufferin Victoria Memorial Hospital and got approval for Bela to take the course. Lady Dufferin Victoria Memorial Hospital, named after the wife of a nineteenth century British Viceroy of India and the former Queen of England, was a Christian hospital for women. The students came from a variety of religious backgrounds, but most of the ward sisters, teachers, and doctors, whether British or Indian, were Christian. The medical staff and the students, as well as the patients, were women.

The daily routine began early for trainees at Lady Dufferin, as the hospital was called by its students. Breakfast was at 6:30 a.m., followed by ward duty at 7:00. In addition to 12 hours of ward duty, the trainees had classes each afternoon, with either a "teaching sister" or a doctor in charge. Later the working hours were shortened to eight hours of ward duty, plus the classes.

Each student was required to deliver 20 babies, in addition to observing a number of other deliveries. The trainees did all the normal deliveries; if they confronted a difficult delivery, a doctor would take over.

Totally unprepared for either classroom lectures or hospital ward training, Bela's determination to succeed and her ability to elicit concern from her friends who helped her with her studies pulled her through. Bela joined several women in the midwifery training program who studied together, helping each other to learn. As she had done at the Bengal Social Service League hostel, Bela made friends at Lady Dufferin, developing relationships that continued through the years.

Anima was one such friend. Now married to Murari Mohon Mukerjee, one of Calcutta's foremost plastic surgeons, Anima invited Bela and me to spend a night with her so that she and Bela could reminisce about their experiences in the midwifery training. A heavy-set, amiable woman, Anima came early one evening with her car and driver to take us first to Lady Dufferin. It was dusk as we arrived at the hospital grounds, but Anima and Bela had no difficulty pointing out the buildings that were familiar to them.

As we drove past the small guardhouse at the gate, Bela and Anima started to giggle like schoolgirls, reminding each other what happened when as students they went out and didn't get back on time. Bela explained to me. "Sometimes when we had a day off we used to go out, taking a pass. Nurse would write in a book, 'yes, you can go out.' We had to leave that book with the gateman. And when we were out we must be back before 6:00. When we came back we collected the book. And if we did not come on time, the gateman would take the book to the matron's office. Then we had to go there to get it, and she used to scold." Bela laughed.

The driver parked the car inside the hospital compound. Anima, Bela, and I went inside the large hospital building that had been both their home and their classrooms for 18 months in 1942-43. In the corridor we met a nurse who told Bela and Anima that a friend who had been in midwifery training with them was working now at Lady Dufferin as a ward sister. Wandering down several hallways and up a flight of stairs we reached the nurses' quarters and found the woman's room.

Sulachana Biswas, the ward sister, answered Anima's knock with an exclamation of amazement as she recognized the two women. "*Yeah, bah-bay*," she shouted. Bela and Anima, standing there grinning, broke into laughter.

Sulachana invited us into her room and motioned us to sit down on her cot. She untied the end of her *sari* and pulled out a key which she used to unlock a tall cupboard. From the cupboard she took out a jar of wrapped candies and gave us each two pieces.

The conversation took off at once. "You used to scold us," Anima said to Sulachana, and Bela agreed. All three women laughed heartily. Bela explained to me. "Sulachana was senior to us, a year ahead of us in her studies," she said. "She was a very good worker on the wards, but she used to scold, oh, she used to scold—because she was senior to us." They all laughed again.

Sulachana told Bela and Anima that Samitra, one of their friends who was studying to be a doctor when they were midwifery students, had later married and left her studies. Anima told Sulachana about another classmate who had died recently. Sulachana hadn't known, and the tone of their conversation was somber for a few minutes.

When Anima and Bela talked about the food for students in the dining hall at Lady Dufferin, their discussion was one of light-hearted complaints. Bela said, "We got tea in a tiny glass."

Anima added, "For breakfast we got a piece of bread that you could see through."

Bela kept it up. "And a banana the size of my finger," she said, holding up her index finger. "That's what we got for breakfast when we were students. If we asked for a little more they wouldn't give it. Only that much we could have." She paused a moment, thinking, then she corrected herself. "That was for tea, really. For breakfast, what did we have? I have forgotten."

Anima remembered. "Porridge," she said. "Porridge, bread and butter. And banana," she added.

Lunch was fish and rice and *dhal* (lentils) and a vegetable curry. "Every day," Bela said. "Except sometimes we had some meat curry. But it was very little they used to give. We used to feel terribly hungry. Quantity was so little."

"Was dinner a bigger meal?" I asked. "No, dinner was just the same. Except *chappati* instead of rice."

Bela, in the years that I knew her, was a very light eater. Had she really been hungry, I wondered, or had she responded as students often do to regimented meal patterns of institutions? Whichever was the case, at the Lady Dufferin Victoria Memorial Hospital Bela experienced, for the first time in her life, a feeling of identification with peers who were her classmates.

Later in the evening, at the Mukerjee house, I asked Anima what memories came to her when she went back today with Bela to Lady Dufferin Memorial Hospital. After their bantering conversation at

Lady Dufferin I was surprised at the seriousness of her answer.

She said that the first thing she remembered was how similar their situations had been. Like Bela, Anima had grown up in a large family in a relative's home—in her case, that of an uncle; her mother, too, was a widow. Unlike Bela, however, Anima had a chance to go to school and had graduated from high school. She said she felt close to Bela because they came from the same kind of home background. "We were very good friends, you know," Anima said. "We looked after each other; we understand each other so well."

Anima remembered that the hospital gave each student six white *saris* with black borders. She had given some of hers to her mother who was too poor to buy new *saris*. Learning what Anima had done, Bela shared her *saris* with Anima. "We washed them ourselves so we managed with fewer *saris*," Bela explained.

The two women were in the same room in the 15-bed dormitory. "We had bed check every night," Bela said. "One of the sisters used to come round to see if we were in bed. I still remember her standing in the room with a light in her hand, during the night."

Bela went on. "Sometimes we used to make tea at night. Anima would say that we had to do the studies late in the night, so we should have some tea. There was so little to eat at meals and we used to get so hungry. We would make tea for ourselves in the ward. That was naughty of us, but we were very hungry at 11:00 o'clock after we came from hospital work."

"Sometimes we would make some *sujee*, (porridge)," Anima said. "We didn't take from the hospital, but we made it in the hospital. We bought the tea and milk ourselves, but we didn't have any separate kitchen or anything for ourselves."

"You did that on the hospital ward?" I asked. "Did you ever get caught?

"Yes," Bela said, "sometimes."

"What happened then?"

"Scolding. We got a scolding from them. We agreed that, yes, we had done wrong." To me, however, Bela justified what they had done. "You know we didn't have much to eat at our meals," she repeated.

There was no social interaction between the students and the hospital staff. Bela and Anima remembered that while they were at Lady Dufferin the matron of the hospital got married, but none of them went to the wedding. "She was a widow, Mrs. Bedford; then she got married—an army man used to come and then they got married—and she became Mrs. Bedford-Finley. We only knew because her name was changed."

I asked Bela and Anima if they had a favorite doctor?

"Yes. Dr. Bhoweli," they agreed, both answering at the same time. "She was very friendly to us," Bela said. "We were terribly afraid of the doctors, you know." The two women broke into laughter. "Dr. Bhoweli was the only one that we used to talk to, or that would talk to us."

There was no provision for counseling students who were having difficulties with their course work. "Anima used to help me study," Bela told me, "because she was 'matric' (had graduated from high school), you know, and I was very poor in my English. I couldn't understand very much, and the classes were in English."

"Were there some parts of the study that were harder than other parts?" I asked Bela.

"The book study," she answered. "I was always afraid that I was going to fail, because I didn't know enough English to do it. I liked the company; I liked the situation; I liked the practical work. I was very happy, except that writing and reading always worried me so much".

Their schedule seemed extremely full. "When did you have time to study?" I asked.

"Actually that was a problem," Bela answered. "We really wanted to do the studying, you know. I used to get terribly worried because I thought, oh dear, when will I get time to study?"

Anima answered my question. "In the night after 10:00."

"That's right," Bela agreed. "After 10:00, we finished everything. Then when everybody else went to sleep, three or four of us used to study together. We used a skeleton to study anatomy. Then we studied with the book. She could tell what was there in the whole book," Bela said, pointing to Anima. "But I couldn't. I had to study harder. I had to study more. She was very good with repeating things; I couldn't do that. But when four of us who were friends used to study together it helped a lot. All four of us passed together."

Lies's plan in arranging for Bela to take the midwifery course in English rather than Bengali was in anticipation of her taking further training to qualify her to be a home health visitor licensed by the city of Calcutta. Even though Bela completed the midwifery course, Dr. Neal, the Superintendent, refused to waive the high school graduation requirement a second time and would not admit Bela into the more advanced course.

After Bela received her midwifery certificate, she returned to the Bengal Social Service League to work with Lies as she had before, doing tasks similar to that of a health visitor, but without the title. Now, however, she had certification of her ability as a midwife. "I was very happy when I finished my midwifery training, because I thought that now I'll always be able to look after myself," she said.

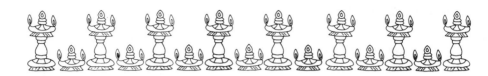

8
JOAN COURT AND
THE FRIENDS SERVICE UNIT

Bela Banerjee and Lies Gompertz worked together at the Bengal Social Service League for nearly ten years, except for the 18 months
when Bela was studying midwifery. Early in 1946 a disagreement developed between Lies and Dr. Dijendranath Moitra, the head of the
institution, which led to Lies's resignation. Typical of her tendency
not to become involved in controversy, Bela did not even know for
sure the nature of the dispute. Nonetheless, she placed her loyalties
with Lies, and within a month or two after Lies left the Bengal Social
Service League, Bela resigned.

Bela returned to Satish's home. After three or four weeks Joan
Court, the British nurse at the Friends Service Unit, invited her to work
in a maternal and child health clinic in another slum area of Calcutta.

Bela had met Joan Court and other members of the Friends Service Unit when they had brought contributions of vitamins and milk
to the clinic at the Bengal Social Service League. Bela remembered
Joan Court's visits especially. "She came to the Social Service League
and saw that I was working in the clinic. She talked to me and observed my work. When she knew I was going to leave, she said,
'Wouldn't you like to work with us?'"

Bela had already known about the Friends in Calcutta when she
had gone with Lies to attend weekly meetings for worship and occasional evening programs at the Friends Centre on Upper Wood Street.
But she had no idea, even when she began to work as an assistant to
Joan Court in June 1946, that she was forming a relationship with
Quakers that would continue for many years and prompt many
changes in her life.

Most of the Friends Unit members lived at the Upper Wood Street
house, but Bela and Joan lived in the neighborhood where they
worked, at the Maternity and Child Welfare Centre of the Sir John
Anderson Health School on Sitaram Ghose Street.

When I visited Joan Court in England, a few days after being with Bela in India, Joan told me about their work together. "There we were, down on Sitaram Ghose Street, on the borderline of the Hindu-Moslem area," she said. "The most serious problem was anemia, of course. But there was a lot of tetanus amongst the babies, too. And a lot of smallpox."

Because smallpox was endemic, they offered smallpox shots to any persons who said they hadn't had one in a year. Then they gave a certificate to show that the person had taken the vaccination. "Bela and I would sit on the pavement outside the Kali temple—the temple for the smallpox goddess—and vaccinate people for smallpox. The people would go and give their gifts at the temple and we would vaccinate them on the way out." To Joan and Bela it seemed a natural, practical way to respond to the people who needed their services.

They worked with both the Moslem and Hindu residents in the area. The community had a high population density. The Moslem families, living in makeshift housing, were extremely poor. The Hindus were middle-class and had more or less permanent housing, but they, too, lived in neighborhoods set along little narrow streets that were extremely congested and noisy.

Most of the Quaker health team's work was with mothers and babies. Joan's interest in maternal and child health in India had started some years before she had opportunity to go to India, when she had read a research report by Jean Orkney and Neale Edwards, two British doctors who were studying maternity standards in Calcutta. The report stated that in some parts of Calcutta the maternal death rate was about 20 per thousand deliveries and the infant death rate 10 times higher. The two doctors had made recommendations to improve the situation.

When Joan came to Calcutta with the Friends Service Unit to do relief work, she met Dr. Orkney and, at her suggestion, found a position in a Red Cross training program, teaching midwifery to students in a health visitor course at the Sir John Anderson Health School. The Friends Service Unit assigned Joan to work at the school.

When Bela joined the unit, she helped in the training program, learning her work by copying Joan as she had copied Lies nearly a decade before, although by this time her ability to understand English made it easier.

Joan and Bela and the health visitor trainees in Joan's classes made prenatal and postnatal visits to both Moslem and Hindu homes and delivered babies in the homes whenever there were no serious health complications. The students participated as a part of their training to become health visitors.

"We took a definite area and visited every family," Joan Court told me. "We tried to get people to attend the prenatal clinic. We just said we wouldn't take anybody unbooked [for delivery]. We had a program of very, very vigorous prenatal care. Unless you got their hemoglobin up, people just died in childbirth. And we didn't have any deaths. Not of mothers."

In the neighborhood visits they went from door to door, explaining at each home that they would be glad to deliver babies in the homes of pregnant women who would come to their clinic for blood tests and nutrition training. At the clinics they took blood samples to test for anemia and other conditions. "People were desperately anemic, partly from hookworm and partly from malaria," Joan told me. "And they were likely to hemorrhage [during delivery]. We tried to get people in better health. We'd go talk to the men. And we talked most to the mother-in-law—did all the appropriate things. Bela and I both were keen on letting people observe their own customs, provided everything was clean."

"We had a lot of tiny babies," Joan continued. "I remember putting them in large woolen operation socks in the winter, because they had nothing to wear—nothing. Of course we also had to give food to the mothers, many of whom were near starvation."

In a 1946 issue of an American Friends Service Committee *Foreign Service Bulletin,* Joan Court described one of the home deliveries after a woman had sent her husband to bring Bela and her to the home.

"He led the way, swinging a kerosene lamp, down Keshab Sen Street where we threaded our way around people sleeping on the pavements and occasional buffalo on the road, down a narrow lane, and up the rickety stairs to Durga's one room which houses two adults and four children. There was no lighting, but they had a wooden bed and a stool.

"We found Durga well advanced in labor. She had bathed, changed into a clean garment and put a jar of water to boil. I could find only one piece of rag for the bed, no mattress or blankets. A helpful neighbor looked after our wants and was not in the way. We boiled our bowls, made Durga a cup of tea and had one with her, and assured the husband that all was well. Within a couple of hours it was, and the neighbor holding the torch rejoiced with us to find the baby a boy."

Both Hindu and Moslem women came to the clinic for meetings that Joan organized to show films for health teaching on malaria and other subjects. "I think we showed Charlie Chaplin, too," Joan said, and went on to explain that part of their purpose was to widen the experiences of the women in seclusion. She said that some of the Moslem women were so poor that two of them would share a *burkha*, the covering garment that custom required them to wear when they were in public. They took turns wearing the *burkha*.

"We didn't have much trouble building up our clientele," Joan said. "Once you deliver one or two babies, you get known." She took only those patients who had received prenatal care from them, and she referred to the nearby hospital any women who were likely to have complications in delivery and those who developed problems during labor.

The clinic was held three mornings a week. On the other mornings Bela and Joan and the health visitor trainees made home visits to provide prenatal and postnatal care for those who had not come to the clinic, to make sure people were taking their medicines and to make preparations for deliveries. "It wasn't customary at that time to have the baby born in the cleanest room in the house," Joan Court said. "So we needed to get people to make everything clean, to boil some rags, and to make sure they had a clean sheet and clean garments."

Joan and Bela also had classes for the indigenous midwives who worked in the area. "There was no reason to dispense with their services," Joan said, "but we tried to get them to wash their feet, because in the traditional method of delivery, the midwives would semi-squat and press their feet against the buttocks of the women giving birth and that gave them firm support. Because there was so much tetanus about from the cowdung, we made little socks for the midwives to wear so their bare feet wouldn't touch the women's buttocks directly."

Joan Court had very high standards of prenatal care, modeled on the London County Council of Domiciliary Midwifery Service where she had worked before going to India. It was to these same high standards that Bela held throughout the years of her work in midwifery and public health.

Joan and Bela carried their midwifery equipment, including drugs to stop hemorrhages, and other supplies such as eyedrops and cotton, in a tin box marked with the red and black star that Quakers use to symbolize their work.

Bela had worked with Joan on Sitaram Ghose Street for several months when, early in 1947, she went to Bihar with Parima Biswas, an Indian co-worker, and Sally and Roger Cartwright, an American couple who were members of the Friends Service Unit. The team was assigned to the village of Ramjanpur, near Patna, for a housing reconstruction project in the aftermath of Hindu-Moslem riots. Bela's work was to relate to the women of the village, "to see the problems of the people," as she put it. "They were homeless under the trees," she said, telling of her attempts to comfort those whose homes had been destroyed during the riots.

During the weeks that the Quaker team was in Ramjanpur, Mahatma Gandhi came to visit Patna. On the day that Gandhi arrived, Bela and Sally had gone in the truck to Patna on business for the unit. When they heard that Gandhi had come, they went to the house where he was staying to deliver a note Sally had written, asking his advice regarding the Friends' work in the area.

Gandhi invited Sally and Bela to meet with him, and they each had a brief visit with him. He asked Bela how she had come in contact with Quakers and whether she liked to work in the villages. He told her he was very happy that they were working in Ramjanpur and that he had great respect for the work of the Quakers.

Bela knew of Gandhi's friendship with Horace Alexander and Hallam Tennyson, both of whom were members of the Friends Unit in Calcutta. Only a month before Bela and Sally met him in Bihar, Gandhi had been in a Bengal village where Joan Court had had an opportunity to meet him also and to join him on his evening walk around the village.

Bela's meeting with Gandhi was short, about twenty minutes, but for her it was a moving experience. That Gandhi took the time to relate to her on a one-to-one basis affected Bela deeply, strengthening her commitment to work with village people through identifying with them—being one with them—whether they were Moslem, Hindu, Brahmo Samaj, or Christian.

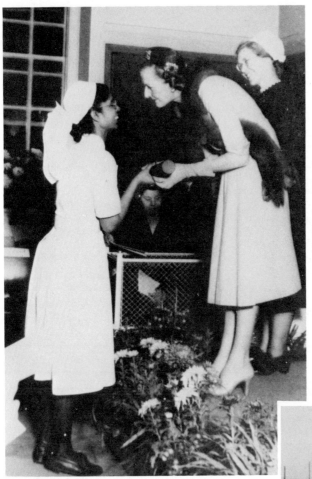

Bela receiving her nursing certificate from Lady Mountbatten at the November 1951 graduation ceremonies, Royal Free Hospital, London.

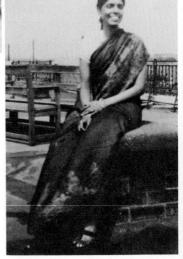

Bela on the roof-top of the Nu[rses']
Home, Royal Free Hospital, L[ondon],
late 1940s or early 1950s.

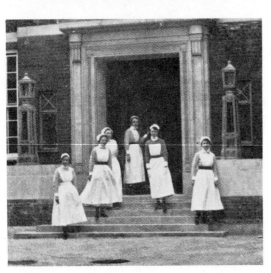

Students at the entrance of the Nurses' Home, Royal Free Hospital, London, late 1940s.

PART THREE:
ENGLAND: NURSING STUDIES

Thou hast made me known to friends whom I knew not. Thou hast given me seats in homes not my own. Thou hast brought the distant near and made a brother of the stranger. . . .

Through birth and death, in this world or in others, wherever thou leadest me it is thou, the same, the one companion of my endless life who ever linkest my heart with bonds of joy to the unfamiliar.

When one knows thee, then alien there is none, then no door is shut.

—Rabindranath Tagore
"Gitanjali LXIII"

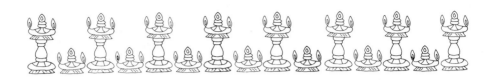

9

TO ENGLAND

As a child in Satish's home, Bela often overheard conversations between Satish or her older nephews and their friends who had traveled to England. Listening to the stories they told, Bela began to daydream. "When I was around 12," Bela told me, I would think about a lot of things, like—I wanted to go to England. I had no money, no education, and nobody to take me or help me to go. But I wanted to go to England. I thought I would like to go and see places there. So I imagined that I could pay for my passage by working on the ship— washing the ship and keeping it clean."

Bela's childhood fantasy of going to England stayed with her during the years that she worked at the Bengal Social Service League. When anyone said they could read palms, Bela would ask, "Can you see if I will get to go to England?"

The palm reader invariably would answer, "Yes, you will go. Your hand is full of the right lines. Yes, you surely will go to England."

Half-believing, Bela would become excited. Then she would say to herself, "But how can I go? I don't know English, and I don't have any place to go."

Telling about it, Bela laughed and said, "I had a hope always, but I never hoped very highly. It was a kind of dream that I used to have."

During the year that she worked with Joan Court, Bela began to dream again when Joan suggested that she should go to London for nurses' training. Bela, remembering her childhood fantasy, showed great enthusiasm. "She had no expectations, really—only dreams," Joan recalled.

Joan Court identified with Bela's daydreams about England; as a child she had looked at the ships on the English coast as they embarked for the orient and imagined that someday she would go to India. "In that sense Bela and I are like sisters," Joan told me. "It's one of those opposites: she wanted to go to England; I wanted to go to India."

Beyond the shared dream, Joan Court had spotted a potential in Bela that she thought should be allowed to develop. "She was bright, intelligent, quick, and dedicated," Joan said in describing Bela. "And I realized that if she didn't get good training, she would be hampered in doing the sort of work she might want to do in the future.

"I could understand that anybody who gets hold of Bela as companion and co-worker will be very reluctant to let her go, because she is lovely to have around," Joan continued, supporting her view by listing some of Bela's qualities that she appreciated: "She takes a lot of responsibility. She cares for whomever she is with. She is interesting."

Joan was afraid she might depend on Bela too much, as she believed Bela's co-workers at the Bengal Social Service League had done. "I thought she was destined for better things," she said.

Although Bela longed to follow Joan's suggestion to go to England for nurses' training, her first reaction was that it would not be possible because of her mother. "My mother is old and is not well, and I am looking after her. It would be difficult for me to leave her," she told Joan. Joan suggested that Bela's mother might go to her other daughter's home while Bela was in England; the members of the Friends unit could provide some financial help.

Joan began to talk about her idea with others at the Friends Centre, and the plans fell quickly into place. "I never thought it would happen quite so soon, actually," Joan said, remembering. "I think I probably paid too little attention to her educational needs, or I would have seen to it she learned more English," she added.

The Friends Service Unit in Calcutta used a grant they had received from Tata Industries in Bombay to pay Bela's ship travel to and from England. Expenses in England were minimal, since the Royal Free Hospital where she was accepted in the nurses' training program provided room and board and a stipend of seven pounds a month for all their students.

The Friends Unit helped make Bela's travel arrangements. Harry Abrahamson, officer-in-charge of the unit, went with Bela when she was having problems with some of the travel papers that were required. "As soon as they saw it was someone from Friends Centre, I had no trouble," Bela remembered.

Joan Court helped her fill out her passport application. Required to state a birthdate, Bela did not know what to do because she did not know when she was born, and her mother could not remember. Joan said that since they were really like sisters anyway, she could have her birthday, and they would be twins. On the passport application, in the blank for 'date of birth,' Bela wrote, "12 April 1919."

When it was definite that Bela would go to England, she spent some time at her sister's home, after moving her mother there. Shortly before she left for England, she moved to the Friends Centre on Upper Wood Street. "Joan kept me there to get me fat," Bela joked. "She said, 'I have to make Bela fat; otherwise they might reject her when she gets to England.' Because I was very, very thin, they thought I needed special food. Bread. Milk. Butter. All those things were special because of the shortages after the war."

During the time she lived at the Friends Centre, Bela became better acquainted with the British and American Quakers who were members of the Friends Service Unit. She appreciated the opportunity to attend the programs that members of the unit presented at the Friends Centre on Saturday evenings. With her earlier interest in the writings of Rabindranath Tagore, she especially enjoyed Hallam Tennyson's programs on poets of the world and Horace Alexander's lectures on world religions.

Margot Tennyson, one of the team members who became Bela's close friend later in England, remembered that during those days when they first met in Calcutta, Bela was extremely shy and spoke very poor English.

When the time came for Bela to leave for England, Harry Abrahamson invited her half brother Satish and her favorite niece Pushbanjali to go along in the jeep when he and others from the Friends Centre took her to the train station. From Calcutta she would travel by train across India to Bombay, where she was to board the ship.

Pushbanjali's memory of the event is vivid. "All those people—the Quakers—they were in such a consoling attitude. My aunt was smiling, and she was in tears. She was running to them and she was running to my father and me—she was sort of shuttling, you know—coming to me, sometimes embracing me, weeping, then smiling. Then she went into the train carriage; she was smiling and weeping at the same time and waving her hands. All these people, and my father and I—we waved back. My father was so moved he was almost in tears. Harry Abrahamson and the other Quakers saw our plight, so they took us to tea in a restaurant on our way back."

Bela had been listening to Pushbanjali's version of the farewell. I asked her what she did after the train left and she was on her way to England. "I cried on the train also," she said. "I cried on the ship."

Except for nearby Bihar, Bela had never been outside the state of Bengal. She was grateful that the Quakers had arranged for someone in Bombay to help her change from the train to the large British passenger ship, *The Empress of Scotland*, on which she was booked for the voyage.

Because the second-class tickets were sold out when she needed to leave in order to reach London by the time her nurses training course started, she had purchased a first-class ticket. She thought of her childhood plan of paying for her journey to England by cleaning the ship, "but instead I had to go by first class."

"I was so seasick," she said. "I had to lie down for about half of the time. And I was glad I didn't need to be washing the ship to pay for my passage."

Because she was seasick and homesick and worried about having left her mother, during the first few days she stayed in her room most of the time. A few times, when she was not too nauseated to eat, she went to the dining room for meals.

About four or five days into the trip she went up to the deck and became ill there. She found a place to lie down and soon an elderly woman came to comfort her, offering her a biscuit (soda cracker) to ease her nausea. The two began to visit; when Bela said her name, the woman became excited. "I've been looking for you since we left Bombay," she said. When members of the Friends Unit in Calcutta had learned that the woman, Mary Allen, a Quaker on her way back to her home in England after a trip to India, would be on *The Empress of Scotland*, they had written to ask her to try to meet Bela.

The remaining two weeks on the ship were more pleasant for Bela, despite her seasickness. As she spent time with Mary Allen and got acquainted with other people at mealtimes in the dining room, the trip went by more rapidly.

The Empress of Scotland docked at Liverpool near the end of April 1947. Ruth and Stephen Lee, who had been on the Quaker team in Calcutta before Bela had worked with Joan Court, met the ship and helped Bela board the train to go on to London. Roderick Ede, who was in charge of the Asia Desk at the Friends Service Council, met her train at Euston Station which was near Friends House, where he took her at once to meet other Quakers who were interested in her association with the Calcutta unit. When classes began a few days after Bela's arrival, Roderick Ede took Bela to the Royal Free Hospital.

Bela had traveled far from her village birthplace, far from her childhood home with Satish's family, far from the clinic work with Lies Gompertz at the Bengal Social Service League. Always immersing herself in the experiences of the moment at each stage of her life,

Bela had lived and worked with a contentment that was not indicative of the changes that her future would hold. Yet each time when the opportunity came for her life to take on a new dimension, she dreamed and saw the dream come true.

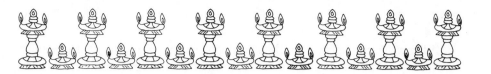

10
NURSES' TRAINING AT
ROYAL FREE HOSPITAL

In May 1947, Bela Banerjee began her studies at London's Royal Free Hospital, where she had been accepted for nurses' training. She quickly became acquainted with other women at the hospital. Although she was slightly older than most of the other nursing students, she made friends easily. "Nurse Collier, nurse Malcolm, nurse McKenzie—these were all friends," Bela told me. "I had so many friends."

Bela's closest friend among the nursing students was Olive Grabham. When I went to England to learn more about Bela's life there, Olive Grabham took me to the Royal Free Hospital where she and Bela had received their nurses' training.

Olive and I walked into the hospital grounds through the main entrance, beneath a sign carved into large yellow brick above the gateway. *"General Hospital,"* it said. We stood just inside the entrance and looked around. The old Royal Free Hospital is a large complex of three- to six-story buildings, covering most of a city block. A new Royal Free Hospital in another part of London has replaced the old hospital, and many of the buildings in the old hospital compound were no longer being used. Nearly all had broken windows. Scattered papers had blown against the run-down structures. "It's pathetic how they've let it go," Olive said.

Founded in 1828 to provide medical care to the poor, the Royal Free Hospital had beds for nearly 500 patients when Bela and Olive were student nurses there. Olive described how crowded the hospital had been then. At that time shortly after World War II, reconstruction had not yet been finished in those parts of the hospital that had been bombed. Although the rubble that we saw did not include any parts from the buildings themselves, it was easy to imagine how it might have looked after the bombings.

We wandered around the empty courtyard until we came to a tunnel that led down and then up again—a walkway between two buildings. After some initial hesitation on my part, Olive and I went laughing into the tunnel, and the sound reverberated against the walls. I asked where the tunnel led and she told me it went to other wards and to the Nurses' Home. "Back then it was kept up nice," she said.

The sound of our footsteps echoed as we walked through the tunnel. I was glad when we came out into another courtyard with tall red brick buildings on either side of us. A sign on one building read, "*Out Patients.*" "These were the maternity wards, all around here," Olive said, as we walked past another abandoned building.

The next building, constructed of a darker red brick than the maternity wards, appeared to be in use; there were curtains at the windows. I guessed it to be an apartment building. "This was the Nurses' Home, where we lived," Olive told me.

The Nurses' Home was six stories tall. All members of the nursing staff had had apartments in the building and each of the 300 or so students had had individual rooms. Classrooms were on the first floor.

As I focused my camera for a picture of the building that had been Bela's home in London, a young couple came out of the door, arm in arm. Olive chuckled softly and, after they passed us, she said, almost in a whisper, "When Bela and I lived here, no young man was allowed to cross the doorway."

After our visit at the old Royal Free Hospital complex, Olive Grabham took me to meet Joan Bocock, who had been the principal tutor at the Royal Free Hospital during most of the time Bela was a student there. Over tea and scones at her flat in the Brixton area of London, Miss Bocock spoke about Bela's problems with her studies and her determination to complete her training.

Bela had great difficulty with her academic studies throughout her nurses' training program. Although the nursing students at the Royal Free came from all over the world, Bela was at a greater disadvantage than most because she had not received basic schooling as a child. With her haphazard education she had never learned, even in her own language, how to pick out important facts from the material she was studying or how to organize her thinking in a logical sequence. According to Miss Bocock, Bela found it very difficult to do systematic study. "It was really sheer perserverance—and great humility, as well—because to go back again and again is not easy,"

Miss Bocock said. "Certainly my memories of her were her determination and her interminable willingness to go on again."

I thought back to what Bela had told me a few days before when she talked about her study in London. "In the beginning I couldn't understand anything. I would go to the classes to get used to it, listening to how they said things, but I couldn't follow the lecture."

Several of Bela's classmates gave her support. Usually two or three of the nursing students studied together, asking questions of one another to review the material, and helping Bela when she found the lessons difficult to understand. "We would do our best to help her see through her problems with her studies," Olive Grabham told me.

Miss Bocock remembered, too. "Everybody came to talk to me about failure and to discuss what we could do," She said with a laugh. "With Bela's background and lack of educational standards, I don't know how she finally achieved her nurses' training, but she did," Joan Bocock said. "I had nothing to do with bringing Bela to the Royal Free, but I helped her stay."

"You gave her extra tutoring?" I asked.

She nodded. "It was not only I. Several of the other teachers helped. Because Bela was always very keen to learn, somehow or other—between us—we managed."

For the first three months after she arrived, Bela went to the lectures that the teaching nurses gave to the nursing students, but she did not take training in the wards. It seemed to Bela there were a lot of lectures.

Then Dame Elizabeth Cockayne, the matron of the hospital, decided to reverse the procedure, omitting the lecture requirement for Bela and having her spend time in the wards, visiting patients and learning to understand both English and hospital procedure in a less structured manner.

Dame Elizabeth was determined to fulfill the obligation to provide training for students who had come from India and other British colonies for their nurses' training, even though it was difficult for the students and the teachers, as well. In Bela's case the soundness of this approach was confirmed to Dame Elizabeth several years later when she learned about Bela's work in India. "I recall being very impressed by the breadth of her work in teaching other workers and patients and in coping with the major problems of India," Dame Elizabeth wrote to me.

Early in her study, Bela took a five-week course in Intermediate English at the Polytechnic Institute in London. "I got a very nice, big certificate from them when I finished," she said, laughing as she compared its size to the small certificate that she later received after completing her nurses' training. Even more impressive was the personal manner in which she was presented with the Polytechnic certificate. "On the 15th August 1947—Independence Day—the teacher brought the certificate to me. She said, "Today is the best day for your India. That's why I came to give you your certificate today."

Although Bela was continually grateful to have the opportunity to study nursing in London, there were times when she became homesick and found life very difficult. Olive Grabham remembered many such occasions, but she said, "Bela did her best to join in with the other students. She didn't try to isolate herself."

Joan Bocock spoke of the concern of Bela's friends. "They were all worried for her. And about the fact that she found the cold difficult. She found the diet difficult. And she found her studies very difficult," Miss Bocock said.

Several of Bela's acquaintances told me of their concern about her adapting to the British climate. Although she did not complain about the cold, they said she always looked cold.

Others talked about her problems with the English diet. "It was difficult enough for people who could eat everything, in those years following the war," one person said, telling about the lack of fresh fruit, vegetables, eggs, and meat, "and for those who couldn't—who were vegetarians or who found the food unappetizing—it could easily have been a deficient diet."

While Bela did not admit to problems most of the time with the climate or the food in England, she did tell me about her difficulties with her studies. Bela was always disappointed when she failed, but determination rather than discouragement was a major characteristic of her personality. According to Joan Bocock, she overcame a lot because of her idealism. "It took a lot of moral courage—all the time," Miss Bocock said, "to cope with all the problems she faced."

After Bela failed her first attempt to take one of the examinations required for her training, Quakers in London asked Charles Lindsay, a professor of linguistics, to tutor her in English. In early January 1949 Bela began visiting the Lindsays' small cottage in Regents Parks for English lessons with Charles. With the next examination only a month away, Charles told his wife Muriel that he did not think he could possibly get Bela's English "up to scratch" in such a short time, but he was ready to try.

After Bela failed her second attempt at the exam, in spite of the concentrated tutoring, Charles Lindsay went to see Joan Bocock. Miss Bocock told Professor Lindsay that Bela's nursing ability and her relationships with patients were excellent, but she pointed out that a nurse must be able to write accurate reports. Nevertheless, the professor persuaded Miss Bocock to give Bela another chance. From then on Bela was a frequent visitor at the Lindsay home.

Joan Bocock was not surprised to see Bela's success in training health workers and working with village people when she went back to India. "I think very often the best teachers are those who have had great trouble," she said. "And in India she's got her own language. And I think it makes a lot of difference if you have your own climate and your own food."

Nearly 20 years after Bela's nurses' training in London, both Joan Bocock and Olive Grabham visited her in India and observed how she had applied her training to the needs of village people in her homeland. Miss Bobcock's earlier view of Bela while she was in nurses' training coincided with what she saw of her work in India. "Bela obviously had an ideal for herself and for her country and for her people," Miss Bocock said. "And I think that that's what gave her the strength to go on."

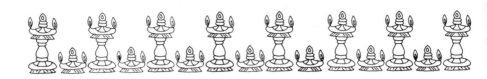

11
FRIENDS IN ENGLAND AND EUROPE

Bela Banerjee's photograph album does not illustrate her life chronologically. Flashes of her life in India and England share pages with photographs of children of her friends in North America and Europe. Pictures placed in any direction on the pages fill all available space.

One picture that appears more than once in Bela's photograph book, as well as in the more orderly albums of several of her friends and relatives, always prompted a story from Bela, accompanied by her laughter as she remembered the occasion of the photograph. It was a snapshot Olive Grabham took of her on the flat roof of the Nurses' Home at the Royal Free Hospital in London. Olive told the same story when she and I toured the hospital grounds together in 1982.

"On the very top, on the roof, Bela and I had our pictures taken," Olive told me, pointing upward and laughing. "Bela had on her *sari*, and I decided I wanted to be rather like an Indian girl, too, so I got into my long housecoat," Olive said. "I often laugh about it, you know." I wished Bela were there to share the remembrance with Olive.

Bela's friendships with the other nurses centered largely around their life at the Nurses' Home. Except for Olive, Bela seldom went home with her fellow nursing students, although she frequently went to the homes of other friends when she had a day off. Sometimes she went home with the maid who cleaned the nursing students' rooms at Royal Free.

Occasionally patients invited Bela to their homes after they were released from the hospital. Generally Bela enjoyed these visits, but once the experience was not altogether pleasant. On that occasion Bela was already asleep when a former patient and her husband arrived at the Nurses' Home unexpectedly and invited her to their home. Bela decided that since they had come for her, she should go. After they trudged through heavy snow, a warm fire in the home felt especially good to Bela, but when everyone went to bed and the fire died down, it was unbearably cold, and Bela could not sleep.

Bela never let her hostess know that she had been cold. Focusing on the intended kindness, she said, "She was so good and wanted me to have a nice time, because she had planned, while she was in the hospital, that when she felt better she wanted to take me to her home." She paused. "In the morning it was all right," she said. Then she added, "but in the night it was very, very shivery."

Two long-term patients, Mrs. Ward and Miss Richard, became fond of Bela. Both blind from diabetes, they could recognize Bela's footsteps, and when she was not on duty they would ask when she was coming. Having learned to knit when they could see, both women had continued the craft after they became blind. Each of them told Bela that they were knitting something for her. Mrs. Ward made a sweater-set for her; Miss Richard was still knitting when they were both transferred to what Bela called the "incurable" hospital. Several weeks later when Bela visited the two women on her day off, the knitting was completed. Bela said, "When I went there, Miss Richard gave me a bed jacket. Though she was blind, she knitted it for me. I still have that," she added.

When Bela had a couple days off from her nurses' training course, she enjoyed going to visit Hetty Budgen, whom she had met at the Friends International House. Hetty's home offered Bela a retreat from the problems of her life as a nursing student, a place where she could forget her worries about her schoolwork. "She always laughed a lot about things," Hetty remembered. "I think she just felt at home and relaxed when she came to me."

"I never saw Bela in her nurse's uniform," Hetty continued. For the most part Bela kept her life at the hospital separate from her other contacts. Hetty never went to the hospital with her, and it was not until a visit Bela made to England more than 30 years later that Hetty met Olive Grabham, Bela's best friend at the Nurses' Home.

"I had just a bed/sitting room with cooking facilities up by Friends House," Hetty said, telling about Bela's first visits to her home. "I had a sort of put-you-up bed to use when she came."

When she visited on weekdays, Bela sometimes went with Hetty to her work at Friends House. Bela learned to know many people at Friends House. On weekend visits she attended the Friends meeting for worship with Hetty.

Bela's visits continued after Hetty moved from her small apartment to a house that she shared with Muriel Trapp, who also became a close friend of Bela's. When I visited Bela in 1982, she was mourning Muriel's recent death as she told me about her friends in England.

Bela didn't arrange her visits with Hetty and Muriel ahead of time. She just came when she had a day off. "Nurses at that time didn't know what their schedules would be very far ahead of time," Hetty told me.

"She always took over all the cooking once she arrived," Hetty said and went on to talk about Bela preparing Indian food. "Finding that I didn't have all the right things for her, she would go and get things—you know, cinnamon sticks and all the different things you put in curries," Hetty remembered. "She preferred having that kind of food because it was a great relief after the food in the hospital. Also she wanted me to like the food, which I did of course," Hetty said.

In order for Bela to see more of Great Britain, Hetty Budgen arranged for her to spend a week's holiday with a friend in Edinburgh, Scotland.

Bela had wanted to go to Scotland to visit the Edinburgh hospital where, years before, Dr. Simpson, the inventor of Simpson forceps that were used throughout the world for delivering babies, had practiced obstetrics.

In planning the trip Bela exhibited a boldness that surprised even herself. She had already purchased a train ticket from London to Edinburgh when she learned that a bus ticket was much less expensive. "Seven pounds by train; two pounds, ten shillings by bus," she remembered. "So I took the train ticket back to get a refund." She laughed. "A funny thing; I would never do it in India."

She told the ticket agent at the train station, "I don't want to go by train. It's terribly expensive."

He argued with her. "But you bought the ticket."

She persisted. "But I want to go by bus, because bus is much cheaper. I didn't know that, so please change my ticket."

Telling the story years later, she still seemed amazed when she said, "and he did it."

When Bela arrived in Edinburgh, Hetty's friend Helen was ill, "too sick to even bother about making arrangements or telling her where anything was," Hetty said. Bela had no problems coping with the situation, however. According to Hetty, "Helen was amazed at having a visitor—especially a visitor from overseas—who just found everything and never asked questions. Bela just looked after her—

produced the right sorts of meals and the right things for her to drink.

"I think that Bela's most outstanding characteristic is her instinctive ability to be able to help people and to single out what they need, not just in nursing, but in other aspects of her relationships," Hetty said, "and to do this with the background she has, the fact that she's had so little herself in her life and wanted so little."

One of Bela's friends in London was Nagen Ganguli, a retired Cambridge University professor and a son-in-law of the poet Rabindranath Tagore. Before she went to London, Bela had heard of Dr. Ganguli from Satish, who knew him through the Brahmo Samaj congregation in Calcutta. Joan Court was also acquainted with Dr. Ganguli. While Joan and Bela were still working together in Calcutta, Joan had taken Bela to Santiniketan to meet Dr. Ganguli's wife, Tagore's daughter Sajanta.

Often on her day off from the nurses' training program at Royal Free Hospital, Bela went to Dr. Ganguli's house to prepare meals for him. Crippled with arthritis, Dr. Ganguli appreciated Bela's visits when they would enjoy an evening meal together. Wanting to do something for her, he said, "I'll send you to Paris for a holiday. I have some very good friends in Paris, and they will be very happy to have you."

Dr. Ganguli wrote to Annuska Rosenberg and Esther Austerveil, two sisters originally from Hungary, to arrange for the visit. He purchased Bela's ticket and gave her money to buy a suitcase, a blanket and other things for the trip. A night journey from London, Bela went to Paris by train, crossing the English channel on a ferry between Dover and Calais.

Bela's friendship with Annuska and Esther was established on her first ten-day trip to Paris, and the visits continued through the years that she lived in England. Esther Austerveil, a nurse, would take Bela with her when she was on duty, and Bela worked with her as a volunteer.

When nursing students at the Royal Free Hospital completed a night duty assignment, they got four or five nights off.

Several times Bela went to Paris on those occasions. Other times she visited Esther and Annuska when she had sick leave. "For a very little thing they used to give me sick leave," Bela remembered. "Because I was so thin, they used to give me more time off." Once she had sick leave because she crushed her finger while helping to move furniture in the ward in order to get ready for Christmas. The doctor "plastered" her finger, then bandaged it and told her to come back in ten days. When he looked at it again, he said, "you need two more weeks." For Bela it was another opportunity to go to Paris and work in the hospital with Esther.

"They were so fond of me. They said I should just come whenever I had time off," Bela said. "Always they would pay for my trip and sometimes buy clothing for me besides," she remembered.

Bela described people with whom she felt particularly close in terms of their "fondness" for her. She used this same phrase in talking about Dr. Ganguli's daughter, Nandita, whom she met when Nandita came to London to visit her father: "Nandita used to think that I was like her own sister," Bela said.

The only child of Tagore's youngest daughter Sajanta, Nandita was married to Krishna Kripalani, India's first ambassador to Brazil. Before joining her husband in Brazil, Nandita stayed in London with her father for about three months. Afterward she came back to London from Brazil several times to visit her father. On each visit she and Bela spent time together.

One evening when Nandita was in England she decided she wanted to see the hospital where Bela worked. Wearing a *sari*, as she always did when she was not on duty, Bela took Nandita to show her the Royal Free Hospital. Having seen Bela only in her nurse's uniform, some of the patients did not recognize her. The next morning when Bela came to work in the wards, some of the patients asked her if she had met the two Indian princesses who had visited the hospital the night before. Bela laughed and told them it was she and her friend whom they had seen.

Another of Bela's acquaintances who provided an opportunity for her to travel was Abdullah Mallik, whom she had know when she worked at the Bengal Social Service League. After independence and partition of India and Pakistan, Dr. Mallik, a Moslem, had left his practice in ophthamology at Campbell Hospital in Calcutta and moved to Karachi, where he became Minister of Labor in the Pakistani government.

In his new position Dr. Mallik represented Pakistan at the International Labor Organization. He wrote to Bela, inviting her to spend a holiday with his family while he was in Geneva for ILO meetings. Never having studied geography, Bela assumed that Geneva was somewhere in England. When she mentioned the invitation to one of her friends, pondering whether she should take time away from her studies to go, the other girl exclaimed, "Oh, how lucky you are that you are invited to go to Switzerland!"

During a two-week holiday in 1948, Bela participated in an International Voluntary Service for Peace work camp in Belgium. Approximately two dozen volunteers from many parts of the world came to the project to clear coal dust from a playground. Bela was assigned to cook for the other volunteers. When it was discovered that the baker and the grocer had given her extra bread and butter—she thought it was because she was wearing a *sari*—the other work campers laughed and said, "We will always send Bela; then we will have more." After that, she did most of the shopping as well as the cooking.

Bela had been in England for several months when Joan Court returned from Calcutta. Joan was at home, sick in bed, when Bela first came to see her. "I think it was snowing and I promptly got pneumonia," Joan told me. "Bela came in with her first snow ball to show me, with her delight. You know her delight in things. . . . We saw each other frequently after that."

Bela must have been overjoyed when Joan returned to England. Joan understood more than most of Bela's other English friends what her life had been like in India.

As other members of the Friends Service Unit in Calcutta returned to England, they provided other homes where Bela could get away from the hospital routine with people who had known her in a different context. Because she delighted in caring for small children, Bela enjoyed especially going to the homes of her friends who had children. Many of her friends included her in their social life, sometimes taking her to the cinema or to see Shakespearean plays. Once at Easter time Joan took Bela to Cambridge to show her the beautiful spring scenery. When the people who had worked in Calcutta had reunions at Friends House in London, Bela was always invited.

When Bela wrote home she mentioned how grateful she was to her friends. Pushbanjali remembered "that used to be a regular feature of her letter—how kind these people are."

Even after she had lived in England for several years and felt accepted by her friends there, Bela never swerved from her goal of acquiring her nursing education so that she could return to India to help her own people. Margot Tennyson, one of the friends Bela visited frequently, was impressed with her determination. Margot said that the most important thing about Bela was that, without considering her own security or future, she was determined to get her nursing training so she could help other people. "I think that's what makes her so outstanding. That's a very rare quality," Margot said.

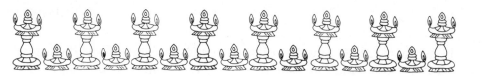

12
HOME TO INDIA AND BACK TO ENGLAND

Bela had been in England for nearly four years when her sister Sushama wrote to say that their mother had broken her hip and it was not healing properly. Bela felt that adequate medical care was not available in Murshidabad where her mother was living with Sushama, so she decided to go back to India and arrange for her mother to be seen by doctors in Calcutta.

Bela knew that her decision to return to India at that point in her studies might prevent her from reaching her goal of becoming a nurse. She had not yet passed the final exam for her nursing certificate, and she did not know whether she would ever be able to pay for her return passage to complete the course. Nevertheless, she felt that she was the only one who could help her mother get proper medical care. As soon as she could make the arrangements, she booked passage to India on *The Jaljawhar*, an Indian passenger ship.

Docking at Bombay, Bela traveled by train across India to Calcutta. Stopping briefly at Satish's home before going to get her mother, Bela learned that Satish and Kripa were having financial difficulties and felt they could not afford to have additional family members to care for. "Where do you plan for your mother to stay?" Kripa asked.

Since she had assumed they would be staying with Satish and Kripa, Bela was uncertain what to do. She went to Sati and Bhupendranath Ghose, where she had gone many times for advice. They invited her to bring her mother to stay in their upstairs room.

For three months Bela and her mother stayed with the Ghoses. Bela got a private nursing job at night and during the day took care of her mother and tried to find a doctor who could treat her mother's broken hip. By the time Bela had come, however, it was too late to mend the break without major surgery. For the rest of her life, Bela's mother was unable to walk.

Bela and her mother continued to express their gratefulness to Satish for his earlier kindnesses. When Satish came to the Ghose's home to visit, Bela's mother often gave him sweets that she had saved for him from what Sati had given her. When she could, Bela helped Satish financially. "My money was for him, because no other people were helping him," Bela explained. "He gave our whole family shelter and food when we were in trouble. So I thought that when he is in trouble, I should do something to help him."

In 1982 Bela and I stayed for several days with Ghoses, in the same house where she and her mother had lived in 1950. The Ghose house is set amidst other lower-middle class, two-family houses and a few small industries and shops along Panditia Lane, where life seems less intense with its narrower streets and less noisy traffic than in many other parts of the city.

One day as Bela and I were walking from Sati and Bhupen's house to a bus stop a few blocks away, we came across a long line of people carrying small shopping bags or baskets, making their way one by one into a small ration shop on a corner. As we stepped off the narrow sidewalk and into the street to go around the line, Bela said, "I used to stand in line here to get sugar and rice for my mother when we lived at Sati's." With coupons, she told me, one could purchase commodities at the ration shop for one-third off the market price.

After three months in Calcutta, Bela began to think about returning to England to complete her nurses' training course, but she worried about how she could provide for her mother's financial needs if she was not earning money. While she had been in England, Calcutta Quakers had helped pay costs of her mother's care, but when she came home those payments were stopped. This problem was solved when Joan Court, who had returned to India to work with the United Nations World Health Organization in Calcutta, offered to help pay Bela's mother's expenses so that Bela could go back to England to finish her training.

Another friend, Amiya, encouraged Bela to return to England and loaned her money for the journey. "She had to go back," Amiya told me. "She had one paper [her final examination] yet to finish."

Bela and I visited Amiya and his family when we were together in 1982. We sat on bamboo mats on the flat roof of their four-story house and looked down on banana trees, coconut palms, and brightly colored flowers in a Calcutta suburb. As we talked, the sun set and the sky gradually turned dark; finally mosquitoes forced us inside.

"I respect you a lot because you helped me," Bela said to Amiya.

He interrupted in an offhand manner. "It is not a question of respect." He turned to me. "I was like her younger brother. It was my duty. And she paid every penny back."

It was not only her close friends who helped Bela get ready to go back to England. While she was in Calcutta to take care of her mother, Bela had asked the goldsmith whose shop was near the Bengal Social Service League to make her a pair of small earrings. When she was ready to return to England, she went to the goldsmith to tell him to keep the earrings for her until she came back again, as she had no money to pay him. Instead of putting the earrings away, the jeweler handed them to Bela and told her to wear them and pay him when she returned home.

Bela went back on a British passenger ship, The *Ranchi*. Her nephew Samiran, going to London to study, was on the same ship. Samiran's memories of Bela on the voyage were vague, except that he remembered she was seasick most of the time.

Samiran's remembrances of Bela after they reached England are clearer. Whenever he went somewhere that Bela was known, people introduced him by saying, "And here is Bela's nephew." Samiran told me, "Once I received a letter addressed to 'Mr. Bela's Nephew.'" He chuckled. "My aunt made a great impact on people."

Bela began to feel the welcome that was expressed on her return even before she reached England, when she received a telegram that the matron at the Royal Free Hospital had sent to the ship saying, "We are very happy that you are coming back to finish your training." As before, Roderick Ede conveyed the interest of Quakers in Bela by meeting her train when she arrived in London.

Bela went back to classes, studying again for the final examination. The General Nursing Council gave her a special dispensation so that she was allowed back into the program after the break, but required her to take an additional three months of training before she took her final examination.

She passed the examination, and on November 29, 1951, she was awarded the Royal Free Hospital Certificate of Training. Lady Mountbatten, wife of the last British Viceroy of India, presented Bela's diploma to her.

It had been four and one-half years since Bela had entered the three-year nursing program. Now she graduated and she wore the nurses' pin with a new sense of accomplishment. Her determination to become a nurse had finally led to her success. Now she was prepared to serve the health needs of her people.

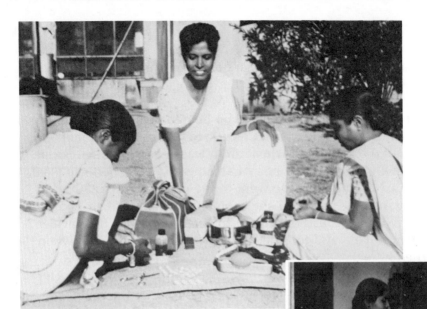

Bela helping health workers stock their
health kits for village work, 1956.

BVS health workers feeding undernour-
ished baby, 1957.

Bela and health workers ready to leave
with supplies from the BVS clinic, 1956.

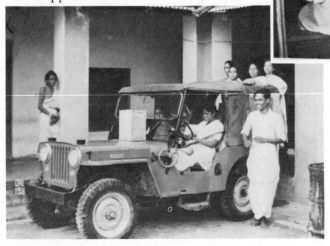

PART FOUR:

WESTERN ORISSA: BARPALI VILLAGE SERVICE

The faith waiting in the heart of a seed
   promises a miracle of life
       which it cannot prove at once.

—Rabindranath Tagore
from *Fireflies*

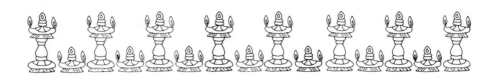

13

RETURNING TO INDIA AS A NURSE

Bela had her nursing degree but no money to pay for her passage back to India: she had already spent the initial travel grant when she had returned home because of her mother's injury the year before. For several months she worked as a ward nurse at the Royal Free Hospital. Then she took a course in domiciliary midwifery at the London Maternity Hospital and worked there as a midwife while she explored various possibilities for work in India.

By the time she had earned money for her travel to return home, Bela had been offered three nursing positions in India. The International Voluntary Service for Peace, who had sponsored the Belgian work camp where she had spent a vacation, the World Health Organization, and the American Friends Service Committee (AFSC) all had openings.

Bela decided to accept the position of nurse at Barpali Village Service, the multipurpose village development project being started by the AFSC in Sambalpur District of Orissa, one of the poorest states in India.

Barpali Village Service (BVS) was designed to relate to the needs of villagers to improve their health, education and economic standards. The project was to be staffed by an international team of Indian and western co-workers who trained village workers to provide extension service in agriculture, public health, community education, and other aspects of development to outlying villages. The only nurse assigned to the project, Bela's job was to assist the western and Indian doctors, particularly in health education, and to train village women to be health workers.

Bela returned home on *The Carthage*, a British passenger ship that took her from London to Bombay, where she arrived on July 18, 1952. On hand to meet her train when she reached Calcutta three days later were her oldest nephew Malay Banerjee, her friend who had financed her trip back to England to finish her nurses' training course, and people from the Friends Centre whom she had known when she worked with Joan Court five years before. Malay took her to the Friends Centre on Upper Wood Street where she planned to live until the Barpali project was ready to begin.

Edwin and Vivien Abbott, medical doctors from Canada who were also assigned to the Barpali Village Service staff, arrived in Calcutta on the same day Bela returned from England. While Ed and Vivien studied at the School of Tropical Medicine in Calcutta, Bela took care of their children—Frances, Billie, and Stevie.

For Bela, the time back in Calcutta gave her a chance to renew acquaintances with her friends and family. Often she spent the day at Satish's home with the three Abbott children, returning to the Friends Centre with the children when it was time for them to have the evening meal with their parents. The Abbott children loved the attention they received from Bela's nieces and nephews.

Bela remembers the atmosphere of friendship at the Friends Centre at Upper Wood Street. The Friends Service Unit members who lived there welcomed Calcutta residents who came to meetings at the center. Quakers and their friends who traveled to Calcutta found hospitality there. "I would like to have a place like that now, where friends could meet together," Bela said, when I visited her in 1982 and she talked about her dreams for her future.

In October 1952, after Ed and Vivien Abbott completed their three month study of tropical medicine and others of the Barpali Village Service team finished their orientation in the Orissa coastal town of Puri, the project members moved to Barpali to begin the ten-year AFSC project in village development. Some of the team lived in tents on the BVS grounds until the buildings were constructed; others stayed a mile from the village in a bungalow built earlier for Orissa government workers. Shortly after the project began, Bela went back to West Bengal to get her mother, and they lived together at the bungalow until her mother's death the following May.

For Bela, as well as for the westerners on the BVS staff, learning the Oriya language was an essential first step to entry into the lives of the villagers with whom they would be working. Some of the staff studied Oriya with a local teacher, but Bela did not join a formal class. For her the best way to learn to speak Oriya was the same way she had learned Bengali as a child, as well as English and Hindi as a teenager—by using the language to communicate with other people at whatever level they could understand one another. Each day she went to village homes to visit the women and children. From the beginning she also became friends with the wives and children of the other members of the BVS technical staff and village workers, most of whom were from Orissa and who, like Barpali village women and children, spoke only Oriya.

Bela's method of learning language was closely related to her philosophy of development. She worked with few preconceived ideas of what she would accomplish. Instead, as she went to the homes, she did whatever there was to do. With intuition coupled with good judgment, she sensed needs and ways to meet those needs that helped her identify closely with villagers and initiate changes they would accept.

Although there were many programs of Barpali Village Service—agriculture, education, village industries, engineering—in addition to the medical program, Bela believed that all the facets of the project intermeshed to help improve villagers' health and living standards.

As the Barpali project developed, certain characteristics set it apart from many other projects in ways that were evident not only to Bela and the other BVS workers but to the villagers also. Bela agreed with the way that Sarat Kanungo, a BVS anthropologist and rural life analyst, described the project. "We tried to build up person-to-person relationships, not only between ourselves and the villagers, but among the villagers themselves," Sarat said. "That is the beginning of community development."

A BVS agriculturist who later worked in training development workers for the Government of Orissa, spoke about the emphasis on community at the Barpali project. "When community development projects forget the community and think only of development, they forget the person," he said. "At Barpali the person was the focus."

Indubhushan Misra, the first BVS educationist, agreed with Sarat. He said, "For the first time, the people talked together about their problems."

Bela Banerjee's association with the American Friends Service Committee at Barpali Village Service opened a new door in her life of service. When that door opened, however, she did not close other doors behind her. With her enlarged capabilities as a trained nurse came increased responsibility. As a part of a small medical staff at the project, the impact of her work was far-reaching, both among patients and health workers. Whether working with them or for them, Bela continued to see other people as members of her own family. Most people responded to her accordingly, and the Barpali project gained acceptance because of her approach to the people with whom she came in contact.

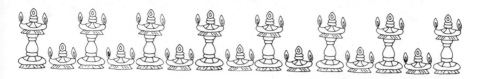

14
BELA IN BARPALI

Barpali is a large village, headquarters for 77 smaller villages that make up the government unit of Barpali Thana. Now the village boasts a train station, a small college, a government home economics training center, a movie theater, a jeep taxi service and a half-dozen cycle rickshaws; when Bela Banerjee joined the other members of the American Friends Service Committee team in Barpali in 1952, none of these features of urban India were present in the area.

On a visit to Barpali with Bela 30 years after she had first gone there to work, these changes were obvious. Just as clear, however, was an awareness of things that had not changed. Foremost among these was the close sense of family that had developed between Bela Banerjee and the villagers of Barpali Thana. Walking with Bela down Barpali village lanes in October 1982, I observed a continuity and depth in her relationships with villagers whom she had known years before.

We were walking along Barpali's main road on our way to visit Bhavani Pradhan, a former BVS village worker who managed a weavers' cooperative that the AFSC project had helped to start. A woman coming from a side street that led to the potter's section of the village stopped us on the road. "*Didi*? (Sister?)" she asked hesitantly. "*Didi*, you have come?"

Bela's appearance had not changed greatly since she had lived in Barpali, although she walked at a slightly slower pace, and her hair, now a little thinner and streaked with gray, was pulled back into a bun instead of being in a braid across the top of her head to frame her face, as she had worn it earlier. She laughed, and the woman knew for certain it was Bela. The questions came like monsoon rain. "When did you come? Where are you staying? How long will you be here?" Then, remembering the Abbott family, the woman asked, "How are Stevie, Billie, Frances, Ed and Vivien?"

We walked on. Bela told me that the woman had been one of her health worker trainees and had been dropped from the program when she became pregnant outside marriage. Bela had continued to befriend the woman and the son who was born to her. "I was hoping I would see her," Bela said to me.

Another woman called out, "Where have you been?"

Bela asked, "Do you remember me?"

"Oh, yes, how can I not remember you?" the woman answered.

Bela turned to me. "This woman used to make bricks at the project," she said, mentioning an experiment designed to improve building construction materials.

"Do you remember Dwight-bhai," Bela said to the woman, giving my husband's name as the villagers called him. The woman nodded, and Bela said, "See, this is Dwight-bhai's wife."

The woman recognized me. "*Yay, ba, ba*," she said, in an expression of surprise that cannot be translated from the Oriya language that she spoke.

As we continued on our way to Bhavani's house, many people called to Bela from their front steps:

"*Namaskar, namaskar,*" they greeted her.

"*Namaste, namaste,*" Bela returned the greetings. By this time there was a crowd of people, mostly women, walking along with us. Some of the women ran up to Bela to hug her; others raised their hands, palms together, in a formal greeting. "I never thought I would see you again," one woman said.

The next one topped that. "Now that I see you, I see the god."

One woman ran home to bring her daughter and granddaughters to see Bela. Bela stopped a moment to admire the granddaughters; she said that the baby looked like its mother whose birth she had attended. The grandmother beamed. "*Didi*, come to my house," she said.

We heard the same invitation repeatedly as we walked along. "Everyone wants to see us. We want to see everybody," Bela responded.

Some people had messages for Bela beyond the greetings and offers of hospitality. "Did you go to my old house?" asked a woman who used to sell *muri* (puffed rice) and peanuts. "Now we have done very well and we are building a new house. My son-in-law and daughter live in the old house," she said.

One woman spoke about Bela having promoted sanitary water-seal latrine slabs as a public health measure. She told Bela that someone had taken the latrine slab that they bought from BVS, and her son-in-law had gone after it and brought it back. "We knew the value of the latrine and didn't want to be without it," she said.

Another woman stopped Bela to tell her that her mother was very ill.

"She is feeling hot," she said to Bela. "You should come, because my mother is your mother, too, and she is lying sick." Sympathetically, Bela asked what was wrong. The woman described the symptoms. "She cannot eat and she cannot sleep very well," she said. "If you would write down a prescription for her, we will buy it," she urged.

Bela had been laughing and joking and shouting to people who called out to her, but when this woman approached and spoke to her seriously, Bela responded immediately with quiet concern in her voice, urging the woman to take her mother to the doctor.

We recognized the temple that was near Bhavani's house, but were uncertain which side street to turn onto. We stopped to ask a woman standing in front of a house how to get to Bhavani's house.

She told us and then asked shyly, "Beladi?"

"Yes. I'm Beladi. *Namaste.*"

The woman smiled. "*Namaskar.*"

Two other women came running up. "I thought it was Beladi," one of them said. She pointed toward the woman with whom she had been talking when we had passed them a moment before and said, "I told her, it looks like Beladi."

In small clusters along the intersecting lanes, people too shy to come up to Bela stood and stared and spoke softly to one another, "Beladidi, Beladi." Bela turned to speak to them.

Passing the house where a village leader had lived during the AFSC project, Bela recognized someone she knew and went over to ask about a mutual friend, only to learn that the friend had died. Again her mood became somber.

When we turned down the narrow side lane to Bhavani's house, most of those who were walking along with us dropped back. A woman stopped Bela to talk about her children; Bela asked her which house was Bhavani's. She pointed to it, and we hurried up the steps.

We had come a half-mile into the village, but it had taken us an hour; perhaps a hundred people or more had called out in friendship, and Bela had responded to each of them. Such was the experience of walking down a village lane with Bela Banerjee.

Bhavani was not at home when we arrived, but we met his wife and other members of his family. A married son lives at home, but a daughter was also there, because it was the time of the *Durga Puja*, a major Hindu holiday. Learning from his wife that Bhavani was planning to leave that afternoon for several days on a business trip, we hurried to the weavers' cooperative where he was working.

We took the shortcut, walking alongside the ponds and then across the *bundhs*, the dikes that separated the rice fields at the edge of the village. Bela told me that when she worked at BVS she used to come past these ponds to go to the village. Often she had met village women carrying their large brass waterpots to get their drinking water at the pond, and she had talked to them about the importance of using safe drinking water from wells with hand pumps. Some of them had justified getting water from the pond by saying to her, unconvincingly, "We will use this water only for cooking; it is not to drink."

One day Bela had been walking beside the pond, approaching a group of women who were dipping water from the pond. They had just filled their brass pots when they glanced up and saw Bela coming along the path. Immediately they poured out the water, hurried back down the path with their empty jugs, and headed for the nearest pump well.

Eventually, as more wells were dug in Barpali and the outlying villages, women more commonly used the pump wells as their source of water, a procedure that Bela was pleased to see had continued in many homes of the area.

In their public health program, BVS project workers had placed similar emphases on drinking water from a covered pump well and on the use of water-seal latrines. Many villagers, however, saw efficacy in pump wells but not latrines. On our visit in 1982, Bela was disappointed to notice that people had been using the fields alongside the *bundhs* instead of sanitary water-seal latrines such as Barpali Village Service had promoted. "I don't like to come here now. It is beautiful, but I can hardly stand the smell," she said.

At the ponds, people were bathing and washing clothes, the women at one place and the men at another. The favorite place to pound the clothes to get them clean was on the cement steps that led down to the large pond beside the temple.

We walked on. I was surprised to see that so much building had taken place between the ponds and the compound where Barpali Village Service had been. It was no longer possible to see the BVS project buildings from the ponds.

We met Bhavani at the weavers' cooperative salesroom. He was extremely busy at the shop because it was the last day that people could get discounts on the *saris* being sold for the *Durga Puja* festivities. He invited us to come to his house a short time later, so we could visit until time for him to leave on his trip.

Taking a different route and meeting another group of Bela's friends, Bela and I made our way back to Dhirendranath and Saki Mund's home where we were staying.

We spoke with Himal Guria on the way. "I'm living just so I can see you," Himal said to Bela and invited her to come to her home. She wanted Bela to look at her granddaughter who had a cough.

"Did you take her to the doctor?" Bela asked.

"No," Himal answered. "My son told me last night that you were here, and I decided I would show her to you first; then I can take her to the doctor if you say to."

Bela told Himal to take her granddaughter to Dr. Mund, and Himal responded, "All right. You said to take her; I'm going to take her." Assured, Himal went on her way.

The day before we had seen Himal's son Shantuni, whose story Bela had told me as we had traveled to Barpali. Shantuni had been born prematurely, and Bela had been able to save his life, though he had weighed only one pound and eleven ounces.

As she greeted Shantuni, whose husky build belied his fragile beginning, Bela acted as though she had not seen him in all the intervening years. Commenting on his muscular arms, she laughed, teasing Shantuni and reminiscing. "Just like a finger were his legs then. How could he grow so big?"

Bela had known Himal for a long time before Shantuni was born, but their relationship had not always been friendly. Himal was a sweets seller in Barpali, with a shop on her front porch along the main street. In the early days of Barpali Village Service, Bela and the Abbotts started a campaign to get the sweets sellers to cover their sticky confections to keep flies from landing on them and spreading disease. Ed Abbott had designed an inexpensive glass cover that the sweets sellers could purchase to cover their wares.

As Bela went from house to house, getting acquainted with villagers, she advised Himal and other sweets sellers to use the new cover to keep flies from their merchandise, but to no avail.

Finally she became impatient. "One day I told Himal not to sell sweets like that, out in the open, you know. It made her angry," Bela said. "But then after a few days she understood, and she became the first of the sweets sellers to use a glass cover for her sweets."

Himal had been married for 16 years when her first baby was

born. Prior to her first pregnancy she had received treatment at the BVS clinic for an illness that had caused her to be sterile. The treatment was successfully followed by a normal pregnancy and delivery, only to have the baby die after six days because of a heart defect. "It was a great shock," Bela remembered. "We were all terribly unhappy about it," she said.

With the next pregnancy Himal did not come to the clinic for prenatal care until she was already in labor, after only seven months. Then she came to the project's back porch, which was set up as an emergency clinic.

Intent on providing care for Himal, Bela ignored the discharge from the woman's uterus, thinking that she was having a miscarriage. "It looked like nothing was there;" Bela explained, "then suddenly we found that it was moving." Immediately Bela and the health workers turned their attention to the tiny infant. "We quickly picked up the baby, cleaned him, cut the cord, wrapped him up to keep him warm, and everything," she said in a rush of words, anticipating the telling of how they kept Shantuni alive.

"Every minute the baby was getting blue and again turning red; we didn't think he would live. We didn't have any incubator or anything, so we made a nice, clean little bed on a hot water bottle and kept him at the back porch clinic." The health workers took turns staying with the baby to give constant care.

"The weather was awfully hot," Bela remembered. "We had no fan, no electricity. We dipped sheets and *saris* into water and hung them on the walls and windows, covering everything, to make the room cooler. And that is the way we kept that child alive."

Twice a day Himal came to extract her milk. Bela kept it cool in a kerosene refrigerator at the clinic. Warming the milk in small amounts, the health workers fed Shantuni every few minutes at first, using an eye dropper. When the baby was three months old, the health workers added a small amount of cereal to the milk. Except for one brief illness which a BVS doctor treated successfully with penicillin, Shantuni grew normally under the care of Bela and her health workers. When he was five months old and weighed four pounds, Himal took him home.

"And that child passed his high school exams and is earning 250 rupees a month now, selling medicine," Bela said, laughing again, as she brought Shantuni's story up to date.

While Bela and I were traveling, we did our laundry by soaking our dirty clothes in a big bucket of water and then scrubbing them by pounding them against a cement floor. After rinsing the clothes in several buckets of fresh water, we hung them on a line to dry. Carefully folding our *saris* and placing them under the thin mattresses on flat wooden beds generally substituted for ironing.

At Dr. Mund's house, where we stayed in Barpali, the clothes disappeared after we had set them to soak and appeared later, clean, dry, and folded, on the bed in the room where we were staying. Almost as soon as our laundry was back in our room, Kusha, a village *dhobi*, or washerman, came to our room, asking if he could take our *saris* and blouses to iron. A couple of days later we stopped by his shop to pick up the clothes. He was working outside, putting finishing touches on my maroon-colored Bengali *sari* with a heavy iron filled with hot charcoal.

We asked, "How much?" and Kusha said, "Nothing." We tried to pay him anyway, but he insisted to Bela, "I wanted to do something for you."

Kusha said to Bela, "When my baby was newborn, you brought rice to its mother. So when Dhiren-bhai's wife told me I could iron for you, I was very, very happy. How can I take money for that?"

Bela remembered when Kusha's child had been very ill and had stayed about ten days at the BVS back-porch clinic for treatment of a high fever and convulsions. Kusha told us proudly that his son is now a *tahsildar*, a government officer who collects village taxes.

Carrying our bundle of freshly ironed *saris* and blouses, we started back to Dhiren's house. Again we were stopped repeatedly by people who wanted to visit with Bela. Both men and women, as they recognized Bela from a distance, shouted out her name and came hurrying to her. Others stood watching us until we caught up to where they were gathered along the village paths, then stepped forward to greet her quietly. Men on bicycles who recognized Bela stopped to walk their bikes alongside us in order to visit with her.

An elderly man stopped her. "Belabai, I look in the paper and never see your name," he joked. "So where have you gone?" Bela told me the man had delivered charcoal for the cooking fire at the AFSC project years ago. Now, he told us, he works at the National Extension Service Block in Barpali. "Today is a lucky day to have seen you," he said to Bela.

A man from the village of Ainthapali told Bela about his son, a baby she had delivered. "He has passed his B.A.," he said proudly.

"Then he got married and had a child. His baby is now two months old."

A woman who had seen Bela on her last trip to Barpali came up to her. "Come, come," she said, motioning us into her house. "Two or three years since I have seen you, and now you've come and my eyes get a wonderful feeling." Bela remembered that the woman's husband had sold milk in the village. She had delivered some of their babies.

Bela wondered what had happened to the high school headmaster whom she had known at the time of the project. "Whenever I have come to Barpali to visit, he has come to see me, but this time we haven't seen him at all." She didn't know his name. "We just called him headmaster. He must be quite old now," she said.

We both thought of Bhagarathi Patnaik, who had died only a year or two before at well past 90 years of age. Mr. Patnaik, after initial opposition to Barpali Village Service, had become the project's most avid supporter among the village leaders when he recognized the close relationship between Quaker and Gandhian approaches to village development. For many years he had come regularly to the BVS staff meeting for worship, a period of silent meditation each morning before work.

Near Dhiren Mund's house on the outskirts of Barpali we met two women, one middle-aged and one probably in her twenties—a mother and daughter. On her head the younger woman carried a bundle of short-handled village brooms that she had made to sell in the market.

Recognizing Bela, the older woman hurried to her and reached down to touch Bela's feet. All the while the woman continued to balance an aluminum pot on her head. Bela raised her up and they embraced. "You are a god" the woman said to Bela. "My daughter was burned, and you made her better. I can never forget you."

The mother lifted up her daughter's *sari* to show us the burn scars on her legs. Her hands, too, were deformed with burn scars. "How many nights you didn't sleep when you looked after my daughter," she said to Bela in a reverent tone of voice.

Bela told me that she had not been alone in caring for the little girl. "David and Miyo took care of her, too, and her mother stayed with her most of the time," she said. The little girl had been burned in an accident in her home when the flame from an oil lamp set fire to her clothing. For four months the child had received treatment at the back porch clinic, where patients generally stayed who required constant care.

One of the many families with whom Bela felt at home in Barpali was the Pandit family who sold homeopathic medicine. The father in the family had been a Sanskrit teacher in the local school during the time of BVS. His sister, whom Bela called Moussee, had been the matron at the BVS health workers' hostel and later became an assistant to Dr. Mund. The Pandit family were among the first to accept several of the innovations BVS promoted in its health program. Primarily this came about because they had been successful in having children after several years of a childless marriage, and they attributed their success to the AFSC project.

After treatment for malaria, which Bela remembered as the cause for their sterility, a little girl was born, whom the parents named Sabita. Sabita was a beautiful baby, Bela said, but while she was still small, she became very ill with repeated convulsions. When the BVS doctors treated that illness successfully as well, Bela said, "They listened to whatever we said."

She continued. "We talked about safe drinking water, so they dug a well and covered it with a pump. We talked about sanitary latrines, and they had one installed behind their house."

Bela and I stopped to visit at the Pandit house on one of our walks around Barpali; all the women of the family came running to greet Bela and the conversation flowed rapidly, as though they had been saving things to share with her.

Moussee said that a couple of years ago her brother had fallen and broken bones in his hand. When he realized that it was broken, he said, "Is Bela here? I wish Bela was here." Another time he had told his sister, "If Bela talks, diseases run away."

Sabita's mother said that if Bela would move back to Barpali, she would build a room just for her, exactly as Bela liked it. "Whole Barpali will be jumping if you come and stay," Moussee said. Everyone in the room agreed.

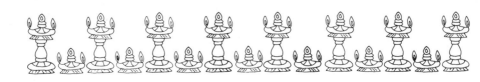

15
MEDICAL WORK IN THE VILLAGES

Beginning with her work as a teenager at the Bengal Social Service League, Bela Banerjee dedicated herself to maternal and child health care of the poor. A new dimension, focusing on a concern for rural villagers, was added to her commitment when she started to work with the American Friends Service Committee at Barpali Village Service in Orissa.

Dhirendranath Mund, a physician who worked with her during the last five years of the ten-year Barpali project, believes that Bela's most important quality is her dedicated service motivation that gives identity to her work. "She could have a job in government service or in other places, instead of coming to a village," he said. "After her training in a foreign country—in England—she could definitely have had a job in hospital nursing or private nursing. Being the type of person she is, she could very easily have made an impact on her employer and gotten good remuneration for the kind of work she does and the way she does it—the affectionate way she makes people feel she is one of them." Dr. Mund summarized his view of Bela's character, saying, "She has really dedicated her life to village people, not looking at employment where she could benefit personally."

Dr. Mund saw Bela's concern for villagers most specifically in her attention to children. "Her care of children, especially the small ones—the premature—was quite more than would be expected from a general nurse," he went on. "She took keen interest, not for money but because of her selfless devotion to the children. Her special concern for the care of children had an effect on the acceptance of the BVS project by the villagers in the Barpali area—they knew that many babies could be saved. After people started having prenatal and postnatal care and sterile deliveries, and became informed about nutrition, maternal mortality and infant mortality was reduced.

"A great change [in health standards] came about because of Bela's influence and her mixing with people as one of the family. Not only the villagers, but also the project staff, Indian or western—many of them feel that Bela is one of their family members," Dr. Mund said.

Barpali villagers expressed the same sentiments. "She is like a family member; she did a lot for us," one man said to me. "The Barpali women did not know how to keep themselves healthy," he continued. "There were a lot of mothers who died, but because of her there is much improvement now. For that, all this area is very much in debt to her."

To Bela, the feeling of family was mutual. When a villager said that Bela had delivered some of his children, she turned to one of them, a young man, and said, "This boy, he is my boy."

Bela's identification with villagers was so nearly absolute that sometimes when a patient died, other BVS staff members who noticed that she was grieving mistook the patient for Bela's relative. Especially when a child died whom she had treated for several days, Bela would become upset and would fast. "I was sad, you know, and couldn't think about eating," she explained, "when I thought about how the mother had so much trouble to have the child and then lost that child."

Totally self-sacrificing when someone was sick, Bela often spent the night without sleep, staying at a patient's bedside. "She was always giving and was always happy when she could fully give of herself," one of the doctors who worked with her remembered. "She did not see it as an imposition; rather it was as if others were rewarding her to give her an opportunity to look after them," he said.

Patients facing emergencies in the night came to her room, sometimes rapping at her window and calling her name in the form that was used for one's sister. "Belabai," they would call out until she awoke. "I am coming," she would answer, and if the person sounded agitated and fearful she would add in a consoling tone, "It will be all right."

Bela Banerjee was the only person who remained on the BVS staff for the entire ten years of the project. During that time she worked with eight different doctors, generally in teams of two or three at a time. Because each doctor had a distinct personality and a different way of working, Bela felt that she learned more from her experience at BVS than at any of the other projects where she worked with only one or two physicians.

Bela's relationship was very close with Edwin and Vivien Abbott, the first doctors on the BVS staff. During the year before Dr. Balabhadra Mahapatra arrived to work with the BVS health team, the Abbotts relied altogether on Bela to establish rapport with the patients, and they looked to her for understanding of the culture that helped them to deal more effectively with the health problems of the people who came to the clinic.

Bela and the health workers developed a system of work that matched the Abbotts' expectations; later they adapted to different methods when new doctors joined the staff. In most cases, the adjustment was not apparent. Bela never allowed any differences to affect her regard for her colleagues. "All the doctors are really very good friends of mine, even now," she said. "They are like my own brothers and sisters."

Although Bela seemed unaware of a problem when she talked to me, some of the doctors associated with the project said that they had found it difficult to fully accept her role in patient care. Bela was needed; they could not have functioned well without her. But at the beginning of their terms some BVS doctors felt uncomfortable because the doctor-nurse relationship which was familiar to them was absent. As time progressed, however, all of the doctors who spoke with me said that they developed close and trusting friendships with Bela.

Bela herself seemed unaware of any problems. As she remembers the clinics, she waited to get instructions from one of the doctors, even when she knew what the doctor would diagnose and prescribe. With the biennial turnover of western doctors and a change of Indian doctors half way through the life of the project, however, situations occasionally arose when no doctor was available; then Bela and the health workers treated simple cases themselves and referred problems to a hospital in another town.

Ralph Victor, one of the doctors at the Barpali project, said that "Bela's strength was her sense of duty and with it a feeling that if she knew the right answers—if it seemed to benefit the patient—she would, without the slightest reluctance, proceed."

Dr. Mund said that when he was at BVS no distinction was made between doctor and nurse roles. "It was a team effort, just a question of caring for the patients."

At one point during the middle years of the Barpali project, there were four doctors on the staff. Thinking she would be needed less at the project, Bela took a leave of absence from BVS to visit Lies Gompertz, with whom she had worked at the Bengal Social Service League in Calcutta.

Lies—married by then to Hugh Seeds, whom she had met at the Calcutta Friends Centre—had moved to New Plymouth, New

Zealand. While Bela stayed with Lies and Hugh, she helped to take care of their three children, because Lies was not well.

Some of Bela's work during her leave was similar to her work at Barpali. For a time she worked in a rest home for the elderly in New Plymouth. She also visited hospitals, both in New Zealand and in Australia, to observe midwifery practices. She was especially influenced by the public health work of True B. King, a woman who had a special concern for the mental health of pregnant women.

When Bela returned to Barpali, she transferred some of King's outlook to the families of her maternity patients. Working particularly with mothers-in-laws, she emphasized the importance of providing an atmosphere that avoided stress and unhappiness for pregnant women in the homes.

Bela also became acquainted with Quakers in Australia and New Zealand, visiting several Friends meetings. She continued to feel the identification with Friends that she had experienced in Calcutta and London, although she never considered joining a meeting. "I believe. That's true. But there is no need to join," she said.

Planned to last for a year, Bela's leave was cut short after six months when she received a cable from Matt Thomson, the BVS project director, asking her to return because the medical staff work load was increasing. Wanting her to arrive as quickly as possible, Matt sent Bela an airline ticket, agreeing to pay the difference in cost between the ship passage and air travel.

Bela had looked forward to the time with Lies because of their close friendship and Lies' guidance in her early work in Calcutta. At the same time, her life had become centered around her work in Barpali, and she was happy to return to the project.

Not only the BVS staff but also villagers of the area were glad that she had come back. Six months before, when the wives of some Barpali weavers had heard that Bela was going on leave, they had brought their concern to Geeta Mazumdar, whose husband Samir worked with their husbands in the Barpali Village Service Weavers' Cooperative. "What will happen to us when Beladi is gone?" they had aked. Geeta had assured them that the doctors would be there, but they responded, "Yes, they will be here, but it won't be the same with Beladi gone." Like many of the other village women, the weavers' wives trusted Bela and could behave normally and talk freely with her.

The BVS medical staff began to see patients on clinic days soon after breakfast at 7:00 a.m. Emergency cases sometimes came even earlier. Usually Bela attended to the emergencies but called the doctor when necessary. "Whenever I called one of the doctors, even in the middle of the night," Bela said, "they always came without any hesitation."

That was a quality they shared with Bela herself. Several of the doctors remembered Bela as a tireless worker. "Even after nights when she had been awake with a patient many times, in the morning she arose as fresh as if she had slept the whole night," Dr. Mund said.

Extremely thin, Bela sometimes appeared frail at first glance, an assumption that was quickly seen to be false when one observed her stamina as she cared for patients. With a calmness that was not easily disturbed, Bela remained very much in control of herself, particularly when she was at work in the clinic. "When others got irritated because they were tired, she did not," a co-worker observed.

One of the BVS directors spoke of Bela's importance to the project. "Bela was always a cheering element at Barpali where frustrations, while not the rule, were often present. We felt her affection and loyalty and expertise," he said. "Hers was a loving concern and service to everyone in need, particularly in moments of crisis." He told about a young worker who was burned while trying to extinguish a fire in the BVS shop. "Bela took charge, radiating a confidence that all would be well, and the rest of us at once became her assistants."

Bela had a singleness of purpose—to bring health to Indian villagers. Her accomplishments in that area seemed beyond her capabilities, given her lack of opportunity as a child.

Early in the life of the Barpali project, women from some castes would not leave their homes to go to the clinic unless they were severely ill. Bela and two health workers often visited the women in their homes, especially when someone in the household was pregnant. Wives of the brass merchants had frequent miscarriages until Bela and the health workers began treating them at home. After successful pregnancies, they became less reticent to have routine prenatal and postnatal care at the clinic.

Bela's role as a hostess that had been a part of her effectiveness in her half-brother's home continued in her life in Orissa. When new staff members arrived at the Barpali project arrived, often it was Bela who served them tea, arranged for their meals, and found ways to make them comfortable in new surroundings. "Bela's presence always seemed to be a happy one," one of her co-workers observed.

A British woman who was housekeeper at the Barpali project for a short term said of Bela, "She was, perhaps, the most down-to-earth worker on the project: no theorizing for her but incessant routine dealing not only with the grim side of poverty, ignorance, and dirt day after day but also with the physical problems arising from unaccustomed community life on the part of westerners in a foreign land. She had learned to understand and be sympathetic to the ways and needs of westerners abroad."

With a sensitivity that crossed cultural boundaries, Bela anticipated needs of both adults and children and found ways to meet the needs. Flowers on the table for the arrival of a new staff member, a can of tomato juice from a seldom-used shelf in the pantry for someone whose choice of the available fresh foods was limited because of illness, a cheery word or a soothing hug for a homesick child—Bela satisfied needs that some individuals were not aware they had until they sensed relief because of her actions.

In many ways Bela was maternal in her association with other members of the BVS staff. An American woman who was on the BVS staff for several years described what she saw as Bela's "care and concern for all of us. She watched over our food and drink, our health and well-being and shared her joys, sorrows, and frustrations with us. She truly loved everyone."

Especially with the health workers she maintained a guardian role. "When anyone had any trouble or fell ill, she would go to Beladi," one of the health workers said.

A young man in the BVS mechanical training program said of Bela, "She does not think of herself, but only of others; she gives everything to others." Other BVS workers were concerned about Bela's lack of care of herself. Indubhushan Misra, who worked in the community education program, said, "She works very hard and eats very little." Geeta Mazumdar, who was BVS housekeeper for several years, agreed. "I used to scold her," Geeta admitted, "because she was not eating properly. Not doing anything but work, work, work all the time. 'One should work, but one should think about oneself, too,' I told her."

When Geeta scolded, Bela would hug her and laugh. Geeta said to me, "Then what can you do? She is like that."

Bill Heusel, another BVS worker, summarized Bela's qualities as he knew her. "First of all, Bela was loyal," he wrote to me. "Whenever she undertook a task, made a friendship, or agreed to work for an organization, she gave it her best. I never heard her criticize anyone.

Through many staff meetings she listened carefully and spoke rarely, discussing problems and issues and not personalities.

"Bela was always eager to be helpful but was unobtrusive in her support and unconcerned about getting credit," he went on. "She was good-hearted and generous to a fault, extremely sensitive and kind. She could take a stand and make her point without any apparent need to win or impress or put anyone else down. Though she gave of herself unstintingly, she seemed restrained enough not to drain her resources to the point of becoming irritable or burned out. She was willing to learn and eager to teach."

Bill Heusel told about his experience with Bela following the death of a patient at BVS after a painful and prolonged delivery. "I was asked to drive the mourners with the body to their village; Bela rode along to interpret. Because the people were too poor to afford fuel for cremation, and because burial was not part of their tradition, I was directed to stop out on the open plain. The body was placed on the ground, there was a brief, agonized outpouring of grief, and then we went our separate ways. Although I'm sure she knew I was troubled over the stark reality of this encounter with death and sorrow, the inherent confidence manifested by her lack of need to explain or justify says something very significant about Bela's character. It is consistent with her apparent lack of any feelings of racism, sexism, religious, political, or philosophical dogmatism. Discrimination of any kind was beneath her dignity."

David Bassett, one of the doctors who worked with Bela at BVS, reinforced Bill Heusel's view. "Bela is an example of an individual who through her whole lifetime has lived simply, responding to needs on an individual basis. She proceeds because she has a good sense of who she is. She is international but local. She has a willingness to direct her life 'as way opened' and a capacity to influence others, notably by the example of her own life. She has warmth, effectiveness and a capacity to mobilize and motivate others that has made possible significant developments of programs in the health area."

Visitors to Barpali Village Service also observed Bela's role in the AFSC project. Lou Schneider, Foreign Service Secretary of the American Friends Service Committee at the time of his visit, said of Bela, "I knew the esteem felt for her by her colleagues. She impressed me as a gentle and unassuming person as well as unswerving in the strength of her commitment to her work and her dedication to the people whom she was serving."

Huston Westover, a Quaker doctor who visited Barpali Village

Service added: "She has a wholly beautiful soul, committed to people, dedicated to highly imaginative and demanding ideals, creative and undismayed by the depth of need she encountered and the size of the steps to be taken. In person and activity she is close to the Quaker ideal. That is the highest praise we can give."

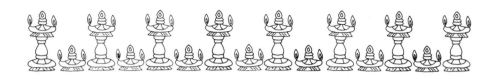

16
TRAINING HEALTH WORKERS

One morning about mid-way during our visit to Barpali, Bela and I joined 19 other passengers—the driver would not leave with less than 12—crammed into a jeep-taxi built for eight, to travel 11 miles to Bargarh. There we planned to meet Kalaboti and Sindukumari, the first health workers whom Bela had trained at Barpali Village Service. In Bargarh, a town of more than 20,000 people, Bela said the name *"Adimata,"* (mother) to a bicycle-rickshaw driver, and he took us directly to the temple for women where Kalaboti and Sindukumari combine religious instruction with occasional advice in maternal and child health care.

Thirty years had passed since Kalaboti, then a young Hindu widow from an influential Brahman family in the Barpali area, had become the first health worker at the newly-begun AFSC project. Intelligent, dignified, and resourceful, Kalaboti opened the way for high-caste women to participate in BVS activities in their villages.

Soon after Kalaboti began to work with Bela and the BVS doctors, she brought her friend Sindukumari and her six small children, the youngest a tiny baby. The two women became health workers in Tulandi, Kalaboti's home village. Three and one-half years later they left BVS to build the temple in Bargarh. By then Bela and the BVS doctors had trained more than a dozen health workers to work in the villages of the area.

Kalaboti was away from home when Bela and I came to the temple. But we visited with Sindukumari, sitting on bamboo mats in a large room where, in the evenings, she held classes in Hindu religious teachings.

Before we left, the wife of Sindukumari's youngest son Sevaram cooked a meal for Bela and me in the family home adjoining the temple. As soon as Bela had eaten the first serving of vegetable curry, Sevaram's wife put another serving on Bela's plate. A light eater, Bela objected. Sindukumari, approving of her daughter-in-law, said to Bela, "When Sevaram was a baby, you served him. You dressed him and fed him. It is right that his wife should serve you now." She paused a moment and then added, "We didn't think then that Sevaram would grow up and marry, and you would come to our house and eat a meal cooked by his wife."

Bela agreed, smiled at Sevaram's wife, and ate her curry.

Sindukumari and Bela carried on an animated conversation about their experiences at BVS. Enumerating what she had been taught, Sindukumari told me almost in one breath how she learned to ride a bicycle, make a latrine, and give injections.

At Bela's request, UNICEF had sent 12 bicycles to BVS for the health workers to use on their village visits. To learn to ride, Sinduku-mari had propped her bicycle against a porch, held on to the porch post as she got onto the bike, pushed against the porch with her foot to start the bike into motion, and rode down a slight incline until she fell off. "I hurt my head when I stopped," she said, "but I was very happy to be able to learn so easily."

Promoting the use of sanitary latrines was part of each health worker's job, but learning to make a latrine was not in the curriculum. Nonetheless, Sindukumari wanted to know how, so Ed Abbott, who had designed the water-seal latrine being manufactured at BVS, helped her construct one.

To Sindukumari, giving medicine injections seemed to symbolize the new experiences that were a part of the relationship that developed between Bela and her health workers. "Beladi showed me how to do it and I did it," Sindukumari said. I heard much the same words from others of Bela's health workers everywhere I met them.

Sindukumari attached great importance to the fact that Bela treated the health workers as though they were her own sisters, not only in their working relationship but in their social life as well. "She didn't just tell us what to do, she did it with us. Talk. Work. Everything we did together. That I liked."

She paused a moment and then spoke again. "Often she used to take us somewhere to have fun also. Not just work only. That we liked very much also. One day we had a picnic, all the health workers and Bela. We went in the jeep, took some food, and ate there."

I had heard of other picnics that Bela had organized, as well as other activities that she had initiated. In general, she had encouraged a light-hearted approach to many day-to-day activities. Despite the seriousness of her work, Bela had a cheerful outlook on life. She saw humor in situations that might have been frustrating for her had she possessed a more solemn disposition. She enjoyed her work and the people with whom she worked. She appreciated a good joke, and she didn't mind when the joke was on her.

Because she had learned both English and Oriya mostly through conversation, Bela frequently made amusing errors in her usage of either language. With tremendous good humor, she enjoyed the repartee that often occurred because of her mistakes.

Once a group of BVS workers were in Sambalpur, the district headquarters town forty miles from Barpali. They had stopped in a local restaurant for a meal. Wanting to set a good example for her health workers, Bela decided to inquire about the cleanliness of the place in a simple way before placing her order. In the Oriya language, she said to the waiter, "Do you have flies?" The waiter's jaw dropped, his eyes widened, and the health workers exploded with laughter. Realizing how her words had been understood, Bela joined in the hilarity until she noticed the discomfiture of the confused waiter and then, between uncontrollable outbursts of merriment, told him what she wanted to eat.

One year during the rainy season some members of the BVS staff members were stung by scorpions and suffered severe pain from the sting. Whenever it happened, Bela showed great compassion and attention until the person's pain subsided.

One morning during this time Bela came to the community breakfast in great excitement and announced that when she had put her shoe on a few minutes before she thought a scorpion hiding there had bit her, but that she had felt no pain. Roy Rosedale, the American agriculturist, teased her. "You were lucky that it only bit you—if it had stung you, it might have hurt." Pretending to be angry, she used the Oriya words to call Roy a bad boy, then laughed at herself.

Kamala Misra was the first of the AFSC technicians' wives to become a health worker. She had come to Barpali in February 1953, where her husband, Indubhushan Misra, was the BVS educationist. An adept seamstress, Kamala sewed for the project workers and their families. When Bela made posters to use in the clinics, Kamala helped with the art work.

As her friendship with Bela developed, Kamala decided she

would like to become a health worker, and she told Bela of her interest. Telling the story to me, Kamala said, "And Beladi told me, 'Yes, you are most welcome.'

"Then I went to my husband," she continued, "and I said, 'Beladi is ready to accept me, so you say yes. You give me permission.'"

She chuckled, remembering what happened. "My husband said, 'No. You take care of the children.'"

Kamala, not easily dissuaded, suggested to her husband that, since all the project workers were staying in one building, it would not be hard to take care of the children and attend the clinic also. "We are all living like one family," she said to Indu. "If one of the children were ill, Beladi is there to take care. So why don't I start the work with her?" Finally Indu was convinced, and Kamala began her training as a health worker the following July.

Rangamoni Patnaik, whose husband Nityananda was a rural life analyst at BVS, soon joined Kamala in the training. The two of them worked in the BVS clinic and in the village of Barpali. Eventually they became Bela's assistants in the training program, with Kamala assigned to the role of senior health worker.

Soon the wives of village workers began to join the ranks of health worker trainees, and other women from nearby villages came for training. By the time Ranga and Kamala had finished their training, 18 classmates had joined them.

In April 1953 Bela visited Joan Court, who was directing a World Health Organization maternal and child health project in Lahore, Pakistan. She paid particular attention to the training program for midwives and health visitors; when she returned to Barpali she incorporated much that she had learned into her own training program for health workers.

At first, BVS trainees had from one to one-and-a-half hours of classes in the afternoons, three or four days a week. They also had training at the clinics all day on Wednesdays and Fridays, with late afternoon classes on those days being devoted to the cases they had seen at the clinic. At that time the training was for six months. Later the period was extended to nine months of training. Monthly refresher courses updated their training. At the conclusion of their training, BVS health workers took the Government of India civil service examination for midwives and received midwifery certificates, in addition to the health worker certificates issued by the American Friends Service Committee medical staff at Barpali Village Service.

Ralph Victor, one of the American doctors at Barpali Village

Service described Bela as "innovative and almost a genius in her training of village women as midwives." He said, "She took women with
strong prejudices about caste—women who often were practically
illiterate—and she taught them hygiene, basic health rules, how to
deal with uneducated villagers; she also trained them in the art of
midwifery." He went on to describe the high recognition the midwifery training program received in the local area.

Developing a health education program in the villages, Bela and
the health workers made house calls and personal contacts and led
small discussion groups. They worked in campaigns to encourage
people to install latrines. They met with parents of school children to
set up school lunch and milk distribution programs. They taught
women to sew. They met with pregnant women and nursing
mothers, telling them, "Feed yourself and you will keep well and your
baby will keep well." Taboos against pregnant and nursing mothers
eating milk and fish were repudiated when the women found that
they and their babies were healthier if they added these protein foods
to their diets.

When Bela accompanied the health workers to the villages, she
drove the jeep, a skill she learned from BVS engineer Bill Heusel because she did not want to inconvenience others to take her to the villages. "Despite little mechanical experience," Bill recalled, "she
attacked the task with determination and finesse, ran the obstacle
courses and fulfilled the requirements as well as anyone."

As health workers completed their training, they were assigned
to groups of two or three villages that were near one another. Like the
village workers, they lived in houses provided for them by one of the
villages where they worked. These homes became demonstration
models, where the workers grew kitchen gardens, installed latrines,
and used safe drinking water from the sealed wells that BVS had
helped the villagers install.

The health worker's role in the villages was mostly to provide
health education, coupled with treatment for simple diarrhea, malaria, and other common health problems. In addition, they went to
homes to deliver babies of women who had received prenatal care. If
complications were expected, or if no health worker worked in their
home village, women would come by bullock cart to the BVS compound for delivery and would return home the next day.

Bela built confidence in her health workers by praising them
when they did well. Kamala Misra and Ranga Patnaik both told me
how Bela had praised them after they had gone to a village home

where they safely delivered twins in an unexpected breech birth. When they returned and told her about their experience, Bela announced to the other health workers, "Everybody, listen, they have done a difficult delivery by themselves."

Each day that the BVS clinic was held, and often the day before, bullock carts would come with patients and their families and would camp along the side of the road under trees, waiting for their turn at the clinic. Emergency cases that came to the project when the regular clinics were not in session were seen in a screened-in verandah that came to be known as the back porch clinic. Both because it opened into Bela's room and because the patients generally asked for her, Bela nearly always provided the primary care for cases at the back porch clinic.

The health workers assisted at the clinics which were held at the Barpali High School hostel, near the project compound. Each week at a general clinic on Fridays and a maternal and child health clinic on Wednesdays, the health workers recorded patients' weight and gave medicines the doctors prescribed. They collected specimens for blood and urine tests and set up slides on the microscope for the doctors to examine. They wrote the reports on each patient as the doctors dictated.

Bela organized the patients, separating them according to their symptoms. After a doctor saw the patients, Bela and the health workers gave instructions about the prescribed medicines and explained about the hygienic aspects of the case, both in terms of treatment and preventing a recurrence.

Generally Bela was gentle and courteous with patients, but she became annoyed and very firm when villagers had been neglectful in their personal hygiene or in the prescribed treatment for an illness. She was a strong advocate of the health principles which she taught to the health workers. "When patients left the clinic they went with the teachings of cleanliness," a health worker said. In cases of malnutrition, Bela taught the health workers to give information about diet and the importance of good nutrition along with treatment.

Sometimes Bela drew on the Hindu religion as a source for her teaching of village women. To reinforce her lessons on the importance of cleanliness at childbirth she would ask expectant mothers who gives them their babies, knowing that the women would say that the babies come from God. Then she would remind them that when they prepare their homes for *pujas*, or worship in the home, they clean the room and the idols and the other objects used in the service, in expectation of the god's presence. "If you don't prepare for the birth of your baby by making everything clean in the same way, how can you expect the god to know that you want the child?" she would ask.

"Bela has very strong convictions about the way conditions in villages should be improved," BVS rural life analyst Sarat Kanungo told me, "and she is a dedicated worker to teach those concepts to others." Sarat, who has worked in the Government of India community development program since the close of the Barpali project observed an important effect of the health worker program that Bela Banerjee developed. "At Barpali, people are more health conscious than anywhere else I have been, and I have had occasion to visit in many states and I have worked in different areas," Sarat said.

"Compared to South India and the villages of West Bengal, Barpali villagers in general and the women in particular are more health conscious than any other area that I have seen. The villages in West Bengal and South India have much higher levels of education than the BVS villages, but the consciousness of health is not there."

Sarat said that BVS health workers had learned a better way to approach people and to explain things simply. "They knew the technical part," Sarat said, "but the most important aspect was their relationship with the people."

Sarat Kanungo is one of several of Bela Banerjee's former coworkers who have pointed out that her impact on the health standards in the Barpali area goes beyond her work as a nurse in a traditional sense. In the minds of many people in the area she epitomized the BVS project as a whole. They, like Bela, saw the agricultural program tied together with improved nutrition, the installation of pump wells and sanitary latrines linked with prevention of communicable disease, and prenatal and postnatal care associated with a decrease in maternal and infant mortality. "Bela is the soul of the whole program," Indubhushan Misra said.

Dhirendranath Mund, the BVS doctor who set up a private practice in Barpali when the project ended, agreed: "Because Bela was involved from the beginning and was there throughout most of the project, she definitely has had more impact on the people than the doctors, none of whom were there throughout the entire ten years," he said. Dr. Mund believes that people in this area still have more concern for maternal and child health care because of Bela's influence in their lives.

About 50 health workers, mostly young women, were trained in the program that Bela Banerjee and the BVS doctors developed. Initially, training was intended for people who would work in the Barpali project; later, women came for training from other institutions and from Government of Orissa community development blocks. Ten years after their training at BVS, most of them were employed as health workers, social workers, nurses, or were in other work related to their BVS training.

Women who took part in the BVS health worker training program were self-assured, interested in the world about them, and effective in caring for their families while at the same time concerned with the needs of others. They remained competent in the many-faceted roles their new independence allowed them to fulfill. Kamala Misra expressed the changes that most of the health workers felt when she said, "My life became different. I was in a bigger circle, a bigger family."

The nutrition training that Bela gave, both to health workers and villagers, was particularly valuable to them. "How to prepare food in such a way that it would be economical and the food value would not be lost—this scientific method of preparing nutritious food at cheap cost was very helpful," a health worker said to me.

Sarajini Sahu, a young bride in the nearby village of Satlama when she joined the BVS health worker program, talked about changes in family relationships that came about because of her health worker training. "When Beladidi came to our village and talked to us about health worker training, my husband and I thought it was a good opportunity for me to learn how to take care of the village people, our neighbors, and our own babies later on. He encouraged me to join the training program.

"My husband's parents both objected at first," she went on, "but my husband had heard good things about the training program, so he convinced them it was okay." After Sarajini's mother-in-law saw how the village women looked up to Sarajini when she delivered their babies, she became proud of her daughter-in-law's service to the village.

The BVS health worker program was planned to provide health care in the villages of Barpali Thana, but the effect has spread far beyond the immediate area where the AFSC project worked. Through the health workers whom she trained, Bela Banerjee's influence has extended to parts of Orissa where she has never lived. In a remote mountain village of Koraput District, a woman and her husband who had been household servants before their BVS health worker and medical clerk training are in charge of a government primary health center. In the Angul ashram for tribal people begun by Malatadevi Chaudhuri while her husband Nabakrishna Chaudhuri was Chief Minister of Orissa, some of the social workers are among the dozen women from the ashram who had health worker training at Barpali. In Padanpur, on the Orissa plains, a BVS health worker is a hospital auxiliary-midwife.

Janaka Babu, the first village worker's wife to become a health worker at Barpali Village Service, runs a clinic in a nearby village which her husband Ananta Ram established for landless farmers as a part of the *Bhoodan* land-gift movement begun by Vinoba Bhave, a Gandhian disciple.

Jagya Pujari, a BVS health worker whose home was in Barpali, is an assistant to a doctor who came to Barpali after the AFSC project ended.

Parboti Giri, a Gandhian worker in the Indian independence movement before she received training as a BVS health worker, now cares for 80 young girls in an orphanage in the hills of western Orissa. At Paikmal, in Sambalpur District, she organized the only orphanage in Orissa for school-age boys. Developed with an agricultural focus to provide vegetables and grain for the children's meals, the institutions operate with minimal outside support.

For a time after the project ended, two health workers whom Bela had trained at BVS—Sarajini Sahu and Kanistha Sahu—continued to work at a Village Health Cooperative that BVS had started in the village of Satlama. When the cooperative disbanded, both Sarajini and Kanistha set up private clinics in their homes. When Bela and I visited them in October 1982, both of them said that they would never have had the courage to start private clinics if it had not been for the earlier encouragement at BVS to do the work in Satlama.

In 1962 a provision had been made for BVS health workers to receive additional training to qualify them for government work when the AFSC project closed. A few years ago, Kuntila Meher, a BVS health worker who entered government service under the plan, received an award from the President of India honoring her as the best woman village worker in all of India. Bhavani Pradhan, a BVS technician who knew Kuntila when she was a health worker at the project, credits Bela for her success. "It was only through the teaching of our

Beladidi and her good relationship with the health workers and with the local people, that this progress has been achieved," he said. Dhiren Mund attributes to Bela the success of the BVS health workers with whom he has stayed in touch. "Where there was a BVS-trained health worker, people would mark the difference," he said. "They could work better than other health workers. They were reliable. The relationship of caring that Bela instilled in her trainees carried on," Dr. Mund said.

Bela and I went to see Samitra Mahapatra our first morning in Barpali. Samitra and her husband Pravakar, who had come to BVS as a village worker in 1953, live in a two-story cement house which they built, not far from the old BVS compound. At the front of the house is a clinic where Samitra sees patients and delivers babies. Beside the house is a large vegetable and flower garden—bright red roses were in bloom at the time of our visit and cabbages were ready to harvest."

Most of Samitra's patients have minor ailments that she can identify and treat. She refers any problems to one of the Barapli doctors. She delivers 20 to 25 babies every month at the clinic. I asked Samitra how many babies she has delivered since she became a health worker more than 25 years ago. She laughed and said she had no idea. "But I remember my first delivery vividly," she said.

"I had taken a leave in the middle of my training, because I was pregnant," she began, telling the story. "We were livng in Satlama where my husband was a village worker. Some villagers came and asked me to attend a delivery case. I had no instruments or other supplies, and I told them my training wasn't completed. But they said I should go anyway. No one else had any training so I went, but I was worried. I just helped the mother get delivery of the child, and it went all right. After my own baby was born, I returned to BVS to complete my training."

About eight trainees had already started their training when Samitra began, along with several of the other wives of village workers. Pravakar had suggested that Samitra take the training. "I thought Bela had good experience and background to teach the women," he said, "and so I encouraged my wife to learn to be a health worker."

Samitra, like others, said that Bela taught her like a mother teaches a daughter, with loving concern and great affection. "We were attracted to her; we were attracted to her teachings, her voice,

everything. Everything I have learned from her—that is what I'm doing now," she added.

After her training Samitra worked as a health worker in Satlama
until Pravakar was assigned to the project headquarters to teach in the
mechanical training program and they moved to the BVS compound.
They continued to live there when the AFSC project closed, because
Pravakar was working with the Rural Industries Project that had
grown out of the BVS mechanical training program.

When people noticed that Samitra was still there where the project had been located, they began to come to the Mahapatra house to
get medical care. Samitra was not planning to take patients or start a
clinic, but after two or three months the number of people coming to
her for help had increased. When officers of the Industries Department would come to see Pravakar, their wives and daughters would
go to the house to consult with Samitra. People from Barpali also
came and asked Samitra to help them with their medical problems.

Samitra and Pravakar talked about what they should do. Since
the Rural Industries Project was a government institution, they didn't
feel it was right to have a private clinic on the premises; they decided
to rent a nearby house, move their residence and open a clinic there
until they could build their own home.

"Just to help the people," Samitra said. "That's how it started."
Just to help the people. What greater summary could one make of the
purpose Bela Banerjee instilled in her pupils and embodied in her
own life.

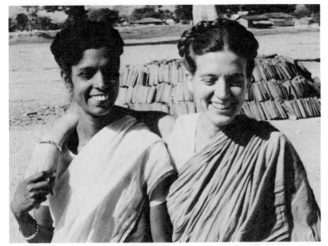

Bela and Dr. Vivien Abbott, Barpali Village Service, early 1950s.

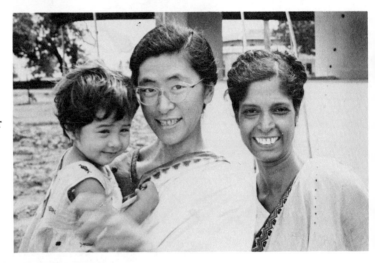

Dr. Miyoko Bassett and her daughter Helen, with Bela at Barpali, 1957.

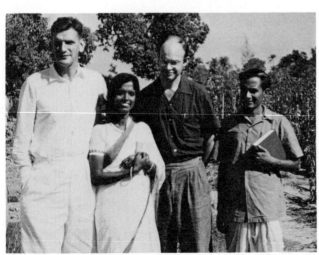

Dr. Ralph Victor, Dr. David Bassett, and Dr. Balabhadra (Shankar) Mahapatra, with Bela at BVS, 1956. (© Westover of Woodstock Photography)

PART FIVE:
TRAVEL AND STUDY

I thought that my voyage had come to its end at the last limit of my power, that the path before me was closed, that provisions were exhausted and the time come to take shelter in a silent obscurity.

But I find that thy will knows no end in me. And when old words die out on the tongue, new melodies break forth from the heart; and where the old tracks are lost, new country is revealed with its wonders.

—Rabindranath Tagore
"Gitanjali XXVII"

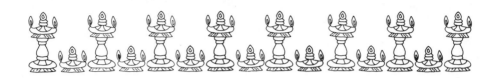

17
PUBLIC HEALTH IN INDIA AND
THE UNITED STATES

Although the clinic at Barpali Village Service filled an obvious need for curative medicine, the project's main focus was on disease prevention. Except in emergency cases that could not be transferred to a hospital, BVS doctors did not perform major surgery. Instead they arranged for patients to receive care either at the nearby Bargarh Hospital, the Medical College Hospital at Burla, 35 miles away, or the *Sewan Bhawan* [Mennonite] Hospital in the village of Jagdeeshpur, about 70 miles from Barpali, in the state of Madhya Pradesh.

In 1961, when Bela needed surgery for a uterine tumor, Dr. Mund suggested she have the surgery done by Joseph J. Duerksen at the Mennonite hospital. "I had taken patients there many times through the years, but when I came as a patient Dr. Duerksen and the nurses were very surprised," she remembered. A Canadian nurse at the Mission Hospital invited Bela to stay in her home before the surgery and for a few days to recuperate after she could leave the hospital. One of the BVS health workers also stayed with her until she was able to travel back to Barpali.

Learning of the operation from friends, Vivien Abbott and her 12-year old son Bill drove to Jagdeeshpur from Rasulia, a Quaker village development project in Madhya Pradesh, where Ed and Vivien were then working. When Bela returned to Barpali, the entire Abbott family came to see her.

Shortly after the Abbotts left, Bela went to Jagdeeshpur for her post-surgery check-up; there she learned that the Abbotts had had a serious car accident on their way back to Rasulia from Barpali and that Ed and Vivien were both injured.

Although she was still recovering from her surgery, Bela was more concerned about the Abbott family than about her own condition. Instead of returning to Barpali after her physical examination was completed, Bela caught the bus for the town of Villai where Ed and Vivien were hospitalized and where the children had been placed in a nursery to be cared for. Bela stayed near the Abbotts for several days, until someone from Rasulia came for the children and she was convinced that Ed and Vivien were receiving adequate care.

Planned for a ten-year period, the Barpali project ended in October 1962. In July, the medical work was phased out. Bela decided to take additional training in public health in a ten-month course developed by the World Health Organization at the School of Tropical Medicine in Calcutta.

After working at Barpali, the field experience in the course was a review for her. "I knew those things already. It made it easy for my examination."

Living in Calcutta again gave Bela an opportunity to renew a close relationship with her half-brother Satish and his family. During the time Bela was studying in the public health course, her sister-in-law Kripa became very ill. While she was semi-conscious, Kripa repeatedly called for Bela. In order to be near, Bela moved to Satish's home to spend the nights with Kripa for the last three weeks before she died.

Near the end of her public health course Bela responded to another family crisis, when an accident occurred in the home of her nephew Samiran. Samiran was practicing medicine in Calcutta at the time; he and his wife Parboti and their baby daughter Lamini were living near the hospital where he worked. While Parboti was cooking one day, her *sari* caught fire and she was critically burned. When he tried to extinguish the fire, Samiran burned his fingers. For two months Parboti was hospitalized. Samiran developed an infection from his burns, and at the same time their baby Lamini had a high fever.

As soon as Bela heard about the accident she began coming to Samiran's home to nurse him and the baby. Her final exam in the public health course was only a few days away, so she brought her books to Samiran's house each night while she took care of him and Lamini. Samiran described the situation. "She was holding the ice pack on Mini's head with one hand and holding her book under the bedlight with the other hand, so that she could read at the same time," he said. "This I will never forget."

Bela's concern did not stop with Samiran and Lamini. Although Parboti was receiving hospital care, Bela thought that someone from the family should be with her in the mornings when she awakened. To accomplish this, Bela made tea at Samiran's house and, even though it was against hospital regulations, carried it in a thermos to the hospital for Parboti. The first morning after the fire she got to the hospital about 4:00 a.m., but could not manage to get in until 6:00 o'clock. On the second morning she failed altogether to slip in unnoticed and finally returned to Samiran's house in tears. "She knew my wife was fond of tea, so she wanted to take it to her," Samiran remembered. "She thought it would give her some relief." Continuing to try each morning as long as Parboti's condition remained critical, Bela repeatedly came to the hospital, slipping in before dawn to bring Parboti a thermos of hot tea.

Parboti Banerjee looked forward to Bela's visits to the hospital. "Although they wouldn't allow anybody to come in to see me during the early morning hours, she managed somehow to bring me the tea," she told me. "She wouldn't say how she got in. It was in the early dawn, still dark, and I was in pain, and she would bring me the hot tea in the flask and she would pour it—I was very fond of tea—and she would talk and console me."

After delivering the tea to Parboti, Bela went to the School of Tropical Medicine for her classes and returned to nurse Samiran and Lamini at night, studying her lessons at the same time. Although she still struggled with studying in English, she passed her exams.

When Bela's course ended, Matt Thomson, who had been director of Barpali Village Service in the mid-1950s, sent her a ticket to come to the United States. Earlier Matt had contacted Bela's friends in the United States and Canada to set up an itinerary for her visit and to collect a "Bela Fund" to finance the trip. Traveling from Calcutta to Boston on *The Jaladhei*, a cargo ship, Bela had a room all to herself. As usual she was seasick whenever the sea was rough. The trip took five weeks, stopping at ports all along the way to load and unload cargo.

Sally Cartwright was one of the first of her old friends whom Bela saw in the United States. Bela did not like to write letters; in the years since she had known Sally Cartwright when they had gone together to meet Mahatma Gandhi in Bihar, she had never written to Sally. But when she was on the way to the United States, she wrote from *The Jaladhei* and mailed the letter in a port. "Suddenly a letter came after 17 years—I was shocked," Sally teased Bela when she met her in New York.

Most of the North Americans with whom Bela had worked, either in Calcutta or Barpali, invited her to their homes. She spent several weeks in eastern Pennsylvania and New Jersey, visiting friends she had known in India and becoming acquainted with the Philadelphia staff of the American Friends Service Committee who had sponsored the Barpali project.

At Haverford, Pennsylvania, Bela stayed with Douglas and Dorothy Steere, AFSC leaders who had visited the Barpali project. Bela was pleased to meet Douglas Steere again because she had been grateful for his interest in the BVS health workers and his willingness to give talks to her class when he came to Barpali.

For a few days Bela stayed at the Quaker study center, Pendle Hill, in Wallingford, Pennsylvania. A highlight of that experience for her was a lecture by a Quaker teacher Howard Brinton in a class on world religions. Remembering the occasion, she quoted Howard Brinton, "All religions come from deep inside."

Bela decided she might want to go to Pendle Hill when she got old. When she was reminded that people of all ages study there, she said, in words reminiscent of the Brahmo Samaj belief that work is worship, "Yes, but I can still be working, not just talk about religion."

When she stayed with Eleanor Eaton, a close friend who had been director of the Barpali project, Bela had an introduction to winter in the United States. She had hung her freshly laundered silk *tussar sari* on the outside line when the temperature was below freezing. "When I went to get my *sari*, I found it was all puckered," Bela said, laughing as she remembered her bewilderment when she saw the change that had taken place in the fabric. "It was all hard. Eleanor told me not to do anything sudden. She said that if I folded it, it would be all broken. It was frozen." She laughed again. "It had frozen dry."

In India, Bela nearly always wore white, but when she traveled abroad her *saris* varied in color and were often made of handloom silk. Bela and her colorful *saris* became indelible memories of many acquaintances during her stay in the U.S. At one home after she laundered her *saris* she laid them out flat on the lawn to dry in the sunshine. "The lined-up colors and the simplicity of the scene—in my mind I see it still," one person wrote to me, using the ancecdote to describe how Bela traveled with only a simple wardrobe of *saris* folded flat in a small suitcase.

When Bela left Pennsylvania, she traveled on a Greyhound bus pass that allowed her unlimited travel—"$99 for 99 days," she said. "For 99 days I just went round and visited everyone."

Matt Thomson arranged for Bela's trip to include a number of study opportunities, including a visit to Community Services at Yellow Springs, Ohio. India was close to the hearts of people from the Yellow Springs Community Services, because of several trips that their founder Arthur Morgan had made to visit Santiniketan, the school begun by the Indian poet Rabindranath Tagore. By the time of Bela's visit, Arthur Morgan had begun to help support Mitraniketan, a village development project in the Indian state of Kerala. Mitraniketan had been started by K. Viswanathan, an idealistic young man who wanted to help improve the living standards in his home village of Vellanad.

The Community Services staff made use of Bela's visit to seek her counsel on a proposal that Viswanathan had made. They invited her to a meeting where the discussion centered around Viswan's request for money to buy a jeep. "Would a jeep be useful for working in India?" they wanted to know. "Yes," Bela said, and she told them about her own experiences driving a jeep in the Orissa countryside when she was working with Barpali Village Service.

As Bela talked to me about being introduced to Arthur Morgan, she showed some of the same sense of reverence as when she talked about meeting Gandhi. "I knew I was meeting a great man, and I felt very happy about it," Bela said of Arthur Morgan.

Before Bela's visit to Yellow Springs ended, Arthur Morgan called for her to see him again. He had been thinking about his dream for what Mitraniketan could become, and he was beginning to plan for a medical center. He asked whether Bela would be interested in implementing such a program when she returned to India.

Bela was undecided. Her major hesitation was due to the fact that the Mitraniketan project in Kerala was a long distance from her family in West Bengal and her friends in Orissa. With nearly a 48-hour journey by train and bus from Calcutta to Vellanad, including a day-long stop-over in Madras, work at Mitraniketan clearly did not lend itself to visiting family and friends. Furthermore, there was the difficulty in learning another new language. Although Bela had learned a Hindi dialect when she worked at the Bengal Social Service League and Oriya when she went to Barpali Village Service, both these languages were Indo-European languages closely related to her native Bengali. Malayalam, the language of Kerala, was an unrelated Dravidian language. Much as she would like to be associated with Arthur Morgan's project in India she could not give him an answer until she had an opportunity to visit Mitraniketan.

From Ohio, Bela continued her bus trip to Iowa, Nebraska, and Kansas, visiting friends she had worked with at Barpali. For our family, as for many others with whom she stayed, Bela's visit proved to be a highlight of accumulated memories. Our small daughter Kamala, a namesake of Bela's friend Kamala Misra, felt an instant link to Bela. While Bela was there, Kamala dressed up in the child's *sari* we had brought home with us before her birth, and Bela taught her to fold her hands in proper Indian greeting fashion and to say *"namaskar"*. Our son, still a baby, responded to Bela's warmth and was soon toddling to her to be picked up and hugged, while he babbled his version of her name, "Bama, Bama."

In Nebraska she visited Bill Heusel, who had been an engineer and mechanic at Barpali Village Service, and who, inspired by the medical program there, had applied to a medical school upon his return home. A physician at the time of Bela's visit, he taught her about the practice of rural medicine in U.S. farming communities.

On her way to the west coast, Bela visited a Hopi Indian reservation in Arizona. She spent about a week at the reservation hospital, observing the maternity wards and learning about the prevalence of tuberculosis and other diseases related to the poverty of the reservation people. For a few days while she was at the reservation, Bela stayed in a hogan with a Hopi woman and her family.

As she went East again on her bus travels, Bela stopped at Pine Mountain Settlement School, an environmental study center in Kentucky, to visit Mary and Burton Rogers, whom she had known when they worked with the Calcutta Friends Unit at the close of World War II. For a month she stayed with Mary and Burton on weekends, while on weekdays she worked at the Frontier Nursing Service in nearby Hyden, Kentucky, helping with the midwifery work in the hospital and assisting a doctor when he performed tubal ligations.

At the Rogers' home, Bela took over the cooking. "I'd come in from work to find her in the kitchen with her *sari* tied back, preparing some good Indian dish from the vegetables in the garden," Mary remembered.

For two weeks Bela worked at the Midwifery Institute at Penn Community Center in Frogmore, South Carolina. In Beaufort, North Carolina, she visited Julia and Harry Abrahamson who had worked with her in the Friends Service Unit in Calcutta and had only recently returned from another AFSC assignment in India at Baroda. While she stayed with the Abrahamsons at the Celo Community in

Beaufort, she met with classes in the midwifery training school for black students. Midwifery students preparing to work in the rural south of the United States heard Bela tell about the work she had done in India to train village girls in midwifery. She felt at home in the rural midwifery schools more than she did in most of the medical programs she visited in the United States because they were more like her work in India than were the large city hospitals.

Bela and I were sitting on a cot in her room at the Kasturba Gandhi Memorial Trust project in the Orissa village of Satyabhamapur when she told me about her 1964 visit to North Carolina. Knowing of Julia Abrahamson's death a few months before my trip to India, I told Bela. "No. No," she protested.

I told her who had given me the information.

"She didn't die," Bela said again.

"I think so."

"Julia? Oh, dear. When I came to North Carolina to see her, she had just come from Baroda. Oh, oh dear. Very good friend, you know."

We were quiet awhile. I had the feeling that she was in touch with the experiences of her friendship with Julia in a way she could never share in words. When she spoke again, it was of something else.

After nine months in the United States, Bela went by ship to London. She wanted to gain some additional experience in midwifery while in London, so she went to Joan Bocock, the principal-tutor at the Royal Free Hospital who made arrangements for her to work at the hospital for ten weeks.

During the time she worked at the hospital, Bela stayed with Millior Braithwaite, a neighbor of Hallam and Margot Tennyson in an attractive neighborhood of old houses with large yards. Mrs. Braithwaite's brick two-story house, was nearly at the top of a hill, above a long flight of stairs winding through her spacious lawn. "Bela was out all day, studying, and just lodged with us," Mrs. Braithwaite told me. "She was a delightful person to have as a house guest, very warm and affectionate. We enjoyed her very much."

After three months in England, Bela spent three weeks in Paris, visiting her friends Annuska Rosenberg and Esther Austerveil and helping again at the hospital where Esther worked. The two sisters continued to be interested in India, Annuska having visited Bela at Barpali. When they learned of the possibility of Bela working at Mitraniketan, they encouraged her to visit the project, giving her the funds to make the trip to Kerala after she returned home.

Bela also visited the Red Cross Hospital for Mothers and Babies in Zurich. "I like their cleanliness," she said. A basket of flour it looked like when they took napkins (diapers) they had just washed and put them in a basket. So beautiful."

Leaving Europe by way of Genoa, Italy in January 1965, Bela made the return trip to India on a British ship, *The Devonia*. She reached Bombay nearly a month later and continued the trip by train to Calcutta.

Soon after she returned to India, Bela visited Mitraniketan for a few days, as she had promised Dr. Morgan she would do. She was pleased with the focus of the project, but she still hesitated to go there to work because it was so far from her family in Calcutta. Instead she accepted a job with the World Council of Churches (WCC) in a refugee camp near the town of Naihati, 35 miles from Calcutta.

At the WCC project she supervised the giving of medicine to a colony of 300 refugees from East Pakistan, all of whom had tuberculosis. The medicine generally prescribed for tuberculosis then was called P.A.S. It was a drug which required a dose of 16 tablets, three times a day. The pills were given to the refugees along with a daily ration of food.

Bela was the first nurse to be assigned to the colony. Her job was to assess the medical aspects of the project. As soon as she went there, she discovered that many people were discarding their medicine each day, because of the inconvenience of having so many tablets to take and because of side effects that sometimes caused stomach upset.

When Bela told the Australian doctor in charge of the project what was happening, he changed the medication, replacing the P.A.S. tablets with streptomycin injections, given every other day. Bela administered the new program, giving streptomycin injections to 150 people every day. In addition, she visited the homes of the refugees to assess their nutritional needs and, as was her custom, to become acquainted with the people among whom she worked.

While she worked at the refugee camp in Naihati, Bela lived in Calcutta in the apartment where Samiran and Parboti had lived before they moved to England. When other members of the WCC team drove a car from Calcutta to Naihati, Bela rode along. More often, she made her daily visits by train, a trip that—in order to be certain of a seat—required the feat of literally jumping onto the train before it stopped in the station. Once aboard, she had a pleasant hour's journey on the Krishnanagar line out of Sealdah Station.

During the year that she was a nurse at the refugee camp, Bela continued to consider Arthur Morgan's suggestion to work at the Mitraniketan project in Kerala. When the World Council of Churches ended their work at Naihati in July 1966, Bela decided to accept Viswanathan's invitation to begin a health center at Mitraniketan, and she made the long move from West Bengal in northeastern India to Kerala in the southwestern part of the country.

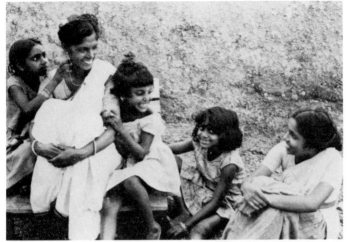

Bela with Mitrani-
ketan school
children and a
health worker,
late 1960s.

Bela, early morning, at Mitraniketan, late 1960s.

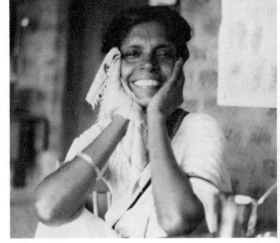

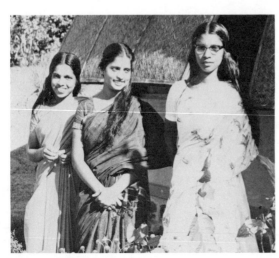

Suvarna, Saraswati, and
Bijoyama—Bela's first health
worker trainees at Mitraniketan, late 1960s.

PART SIX:

KERALA AND MADHYA PRADESH: VILLAGE WORK

*Each rose that comes brings me greetings
    from the Rose of an eternal spring.
God honours me when I work,
    He loves me when I sing.*

—Rabindranath Tagore
from *Fireflies*

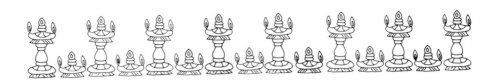

18

THE MITRANIKETAN PROJECT

Mitraniketan was celebrating its 25th anniversary during the week that Bela Banerjee and I visited the project. A welcoming crepe-paper banner festooned the entrance. Loud-speakers blared out recorded music to greet buses filled with school children on field trips and college students on study tours who had come to see the exhibitions at the celebration.

Bela and I had come by train to Trivandrum, 25 miles from Mitraniketan. Sayshee, a Mitraniketan employee who had been a teenager studying English when Bela had worked at the project, met us at the station and took us to the guest house that Mitraniketan owns in the city. Formerly a palace built by a *raja* for his wife, the guest house contains the original furniture, brass pots, and pictures that belonged to the *raja's* wife. As we drank tea and ate spicy deep-fried lentil balls, Bela and I examined our surroundings that depicted a royal past in which we felt oddly out-of-place, dressed as we were in wrinkled cotton *saris* after a night traveling third-class on the train.

Refreshed by the tea, we left Trivandrum in the Mitraniketan car, stopping only once along the road for Sayshee to buy large red bananas that he gave to Bela. The hour's journey through mountainous terrain went quickly. As we sped by plots of tapioca and bananas and the homes of village farmers, Sayshee brought Bela up to date in excited conversation about her acquaintances whom she had lost track of in the two years since she had last visited the project.

As soon as we reached Mitraniketan, Bela shared her recognition of the places we walked past. "This was my health center," she said, pointing to a red brick octagonal building. The front yard was planted to tapioca. "My health workers had a vegetable garden there," she said.

"Oh, I want to see if there is jackfruit growing on my jackfruit tree," she exclaimed, as we walked around the health center. She laughed and told me, "The jackfruit tree grew up out of the compost pile."

When we met people she knew, there emerged a ritual of greeting. A glance. A spark of recognition. A pause of uncertainty. Soft laughter from Bela. Then mutual shouts of joy, and the conversation began to flow.

She joked with the young people who had grown up since she knew them as students in the Mitraniketan school. "Too fat," she accused one young man. To another she pointed, laughed, and exclaimed, "Moustache."

Some of Bela's friends brought their small children to meet her. "This is Sita? Oh, she is so big."

We met a teenager whose life Bela had saved at birth in a difficult delivery. "This is Neesha, my own daughter," Bela said to me. The girl's mother beamed.

The reminiscences continued at mealtimes. "I used to miss *dosa*," Bela said at breakfast our first morning at Mitraniketan. Someone had just brought a second helping of *dosa*, (lentil patties, slightly fermented before cooking and then served cold in yogurt). Bela accepted it eagerly, enjoying the opportunity to eat South Indian food again. She liked the food in Kerala and told me that nutritious food was easier to get there than in some other parts of India. "Nearly everyone grows coconuts and tapioca, and they sell some coconuts to buy fish," she said.

Mitraniketan brochures describe Viswanathan as "a young visionary" at the time he began the project on his parents' property in his home village of Vellanad. Originally he planned only to promote handicrafts to provide additional income for villagers, but as his ideas evolved into a holistic approach to village development, he soon included improved agriculture and children's education as major elements of his plan.

Like Bela, Viswan believed in starting small, from where they were, and allowing big changes. After studying at Santiniketan, Rabindranath Tagore's school in West Bengal, Viswan had spent several years in the United States, both at Pendle Hill, the Quaker study center in Pennsylvania, and with Arthur Morgan at Community Services in Yellow Springs, Ohio. He also had been an observer of the Danish folk-school movement for several months. Finally, having developed his ideas into a workable format, he had returned to India in 1957 to begin his work at Mitraniketan.

Viswan is soft-spoken, almost always smiling. Although sometimes he gives the impression of being far away in his thoughts, he has a charisma that draws people to him. When he started Mitraniketan, Viswan contacted village boys to work with him to make a road and build a house. "All of them came to help him, because everybody liked Viswan very much, and he was very fond of all the villagers," Bela said.

Viswan's parents encouraged him in his efforts to establish Mitraniketan. His father, a contractor, designed the first buildings for the project and donated their family home. His mother cooked meals for the people who worked there. After he was married, his wife Sethu, whose practicality balances Viswan's idealism, became the business manager. Viswan's brothers also participated from the beginning, one managing the agricultural work at Mitraniketan, another the printing press, and a third working as project treasurer.

According to Bela, Viswan has an ability to draw on the talents and inspiration of others. "He takes good ideas from everybody. He gave jobs immediately to almost anybody who would come to Mitraniketan. "Yes, come, join me," he would say, never thinking about where he was going to get the money to pay them," Bela said.

Bela was one of the few people with whom Viswan could share his dreams for Mitraniketan at a deep level. "It is always good to have a person of kindred spirit to share, to exchange ideas—to be sure of your own actions," Viswan told me. "She was very helpful in that way. She was atuned to what I was doing."

Bela had a reciprocal relationship with Viswan. "I was very happy to work with him," she said. "Whatever I suggested, he usually gave me the facility immediately. It was easy to work with him."

During most of the years that Bela worked at Mitraniketan, the project was coalesced by a sense of community among the Viswanathan family, the children who attended the Mitraniketan school, the workers in the various programs, and many neighbors. Each morning the entire community worked at various chores together—getting water, gardening, cleaning the yard, scrubbing the room where meals were eaten, washing vegetables for the noon meal. On Saturday afternoons they met informally for recreation; the children learned to dance and sing for their own enjoyment. On Saturday evenings all the workers of the community—the farmers, the health workers, the teachers—met to decide directions for the project as a whole.

The project expanded during the first five years after Bela came. "Pottery. Dairy. Bakery. Poultry. Carpentry. Agriculture. Printing press. Weaving. All around there was something going on," Bela said.

Bela encouraged her health workers to help out when there were extra duties in some other department. "When the printing press had a lot of orders, our girls went the whole night to help there. If somebody working with the poultry project was sick, our girls used to go and feed the chickens," Bela told me.

Bela wanted her health workers to be well-rounded in their abilities. Besides encouraging them to gain experience in the various facets of work at Mitraniketan, she encouraged them to take typing classes that were available in the nearby village of Vellanad.

For the women who worked at the weaving center, Bela organized classes in hygiene, sanitation, and nutrition during their lunch break. Sometimes she had cooking demonstrations, putting together simple combinations such as vegetables, *dhal*, and rice to make nutritious meals and then serving the women what she had prepared.

Laborers in the Vellanad area knew Bela well. Whenever they had a job to do at Mitraniketan, Bela would come to them while they were cooking their rice, bringing *sag* and *dhal* (a green leafy vegetable and a lentil) which she had spiced with black pepper, and serve it to them. At the same time she gave them a lesson in nutrition, explaining that the combination provided a balanced meal.

On one occasion the young men and boys at Mitraniketan were digging a pond for the village. Each day Bela and the health workers boiled tapioca and made coffee for them so the workers could have a lunch when they completed their work. Bela told me a story about the arrangement. "One day I came in while they were sitting there after eating a big pot of tapioca, and I asked how much of the pond they had finished digging," she said. One of the men responded to her question: "Digging tank is not much done, but tapioca is all finished."

Bela laughed, remembering the occasion, and then summarized her attitude about working at Mitraniketan. "It was fun also—happy work."

Anna Glazebrook, nicknamed Roo, was a young British woman whom Viswan met when she was working with a voluntary service organization in Bangalore. Viswan invited her to come to Mitraniketan to teach English at the school. She also taught an informal English class to Bela's health workers and to three teenage boys who worked at the project.

Bela participated in the classes, finding it a good opportunity to practice Malayalam, as well as to learn more English herself. Roo enjoyed having Bela come to the English classes; the two of them had fun demonstrating the meanings of words. Once someone in the class didn't know what the word "chasing" meant, so Bela and Roo started chasing one another around the room.

Roo admired the setting for her English classes. One of three "sort of round buildings—mud walls, thatched roofs, open at the sides, in amongst a field of pineapples," she said, describing Mitraniketan as she remembered the project, when I met her in England. "No electricity at Mitraniketan then either. They would all come with their lanterns. It was lovely."

Roo's room was also in the health center, near Bela's quarters, and the two women quickly became friends. "Bela was very motherly to me," Roo said. "Every morning the first thing I remember when I woke up would be Bela's voice saying, 'Coffee, coffee, coffee.' And she would bring me my cup of coffee in a steel beaker. Always, without fail, she would bring it to me in bed."

Caroline Balderston, who roomed with Roo on the health center verandah, remembered Bela's early morning ritual, too. "She was always dressed in a clean *sari*, with her hair brushed, and had started her day long before I got up," Caroline said. Caroline also experienced Bela's mothering influence, especially when her own mother died in the United States while she was at Mitraniketan.

When David Parry, a young man from England on his way to Australia, stopped at Mitraniketan to visit and decided to stay on at the project after he met Caroline, Bela was delighted. When Roo left the project, David took her place as an English teacher and, before long, he and Caroline were married.

Another person who felt Bela's motherly concern was K. V. Pillai, who came to Mitraniketan as a young teacher and social worker soon after Bela had started the health program at the project. When Bela and I visited Mitranketan, Pillai told me how he had gone to Bela for advice because he was frequently ill. Bela sensed that he was very unsettled and uncertain what he wanted to do with his life; she suggested gently that perhaps he ought to get married. Pillai grinned broadly as he delivered the punch line to his story. "So I married her health worker," he said.

We were visiting in the parental home of Pillai's wife Saraswati, whom I had already met; their children were playing nearby. Pillai stopped talking and showed us a family picture that he took from a shelf in the room. Bela teased Pillai, pointing to the picture. "You should give me one. It is not only your family; it is my family, too."

He laughed but was not deterred in his praise. "Bela is the only person who guided me to show the way to live. My father and mother talked about settling down, and they worried about me, but Bela gave me guidance. She is the prime adviser and friend to me. She helped me to have a settled life," he said.

When I met Mrs. Ammal, another teacher at the Mitraniketan school, I noticed at once that she and Bela called each other "chechi," the Malayalam word for sister. As the conversation developed it became clear that the word described their relationship and was not merely a title.

Bela and I visited with Mrs. Ammal at her brick home on land that adjoins the Mitraniketan property. Mrs. Ammal had first come to the project in 1970 to visit the school when she was employed by the Kerala government as a district education organizer.

"Miss Bela Banerjee was here as a worker," Mrs. Ammal said to me in precise and formal English. "She actually attracted me very much, because of her sociable nature. She was very loving, even to a pure stranger. I had nothing to do with the social work here and nothing to do with health. But even then I found her as a very nice friend."

Impressed by Mitraniketan, Mrs. Ammal decided to enroll her son in the school. Two years later she took leave from government service to become a teacher at the Mitraniketan school. She helped to arrange the health classes that Bela and the health workers held at each grade level and she worked with Bela in visiting the nearby tribal colonies. "Health and education always go together," she explained in describing their work.

"It was very pleasant to work with Bela," Mrs. Ammal went on. "She became a very close friend of mine. Even now when she comes I feel that one of my own sisters has come here."

Bela's sense of family was not limited to other workers at the Mitraniketan project. One of her closest friends was an elderly woman who lived in a small white-washed earthen house on village land that bordered the Mitraniketan health center. On our first morning at Mitraniketan we set out to visit Bela's friends; as we walked along the well-worn path that linked the old woman's house to the project, Bela told me about her neighbor.

Widowed for several years by the time Bela knew her, the old woman lived alone. Although she was poor, she frequently would cook extra food to share with Bela when they were neighbors.

The woman had heard Bela's voice and was at the door to greet her when we arrived. She nodded to me and to Shanta, Bela's health worker who was with us, and then ignored us to plunge into an animated conversation with Bela. At the door all three of us slipped our feet out of our *chappals*, our Indian sandals, and entered the house. The woman motioned Shanta and me to a board bed to sit down, then called Bela to go with her to the kitchen. From the kitchen doorway Bela interpreted both sides of their conversation to me. I marvelled again how Bela was able to switch languages with such ease.

"Often in the night I dream of you," the old woman said to Bela. "Now I feel bad, because I won't see you again for a long time."

It must have occurred to her suddenly that perhaps Bela was staying this time, because she quickly asked, "Are you going to stay or are you going away from this place?" Without waiting for Bela to answer, she added, "You must come here. Don't go away."

Bela came back into the room to sit beside Shanta and me on the bed. She told us that earlier the woman had said that Bela could live on her land and she would take care of her. Bela said thoughtfully, "She had very little, yet she still used to bring something to me."

The woman had been quite ill just before Bela had visited on her trip to Mitraniketan two years before. She told Bela, "When I was very ill I thought I wouldn't see you again."

Now she was feeling well. "I have no problem now. I have my pension, because my husband was a cook in a government hospital. I have land and grow some tapioca."

She directed her words to all three of us: "On the stove there is some rice. Would you like to eat some rice?"

We declined, but had tea, for which she had started boiling the water as soon as we had arrived. We drank out of brass glasses, but because she had only two glasses Shanta waited until I had finished drinking my tea and then used the same glass.

As we left, the old woman said to Bela, "You must stay here. That would be good for everyone if you stay here."

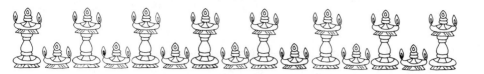

19

HEALTH WORKERS AT MITRANIKETAN

Until Bela came to Mitraniketan in July 1966, the project had no health program. When Arthur Morgan had interviewed Bela in Ohio two years before, he had encouraged her to begin such a program under Community Services sponsorship, realizing perhaps how well Bela's philosophy of public health work would mesh with Viswanathan's development goals.

"I wanted to give shape to the health program, because health is also an integral part of the whole development," Viswan said. "Without health you can't do anything. And the health also should not be merely cure, starting a dispensary and so forth, but total health." He continued, "So I was fortunate to have Bela, because she also believes that prevention is better than curing."

Bela had expressed her aim in her work at Mitraniketan in holistic terms as well. "A public health nurse should think about the whole of the community where she is working, not just one family or one area," she told me. "I thought that was the best way I could help. I could work with the individual, family, and community, too."

For the first year of the Mitraniketan health program, there was no doctor. Local doctors cooperated when Bela sought their advice. When a patient needed blood analysis or hospital care, she arranged for those services at a hospital in the nearby city of Trivandrum. In 1967 Jean Kohler, an American doctor, was assigned to Mitraniketan. Since then several doctors have been associated with the project, most of them, except for Dr. Kohler, commuting to Mitraniketan to see patients at the clinic as a supplement to a medical practice in other nearby areas.

Bela began her work at Mitraniketan in the same way she had in Calcutta and Barpali—by visiting homes in the area to become acquainted with people and to learn the language. Even though Bela did not learn to speak fluent Malayalam, she was very good at communicating with people. Her good-natured attempts at speaking the language in the local dialect, accompanied by gestures, and a readiness to laugh at her own mistakes, endeared her to the families whom she visited. Gradually, as she became acquainted with a family, she introduced her ideas of nutrition, sanitation, and family planning.

One co-worker said of Bela, "She introduced the health program through persuasion, education, training, and close affection."

A British worker at the project who sometimes accompanied Bela on her home visits described Bela's approach to family planning. "She would look at the family, she'd look at all the children, and she'd admire them and the new baby. And then she would look at the mother, or the father if he was there, and she'd say, '*madi*?' which means 'enough?' and then, quite firmly, she would repeat, 'Yes, enough. You have a very nice family.'"

Among Bela's friends in the village of Vellanad were three girls—Suvarna, Saraswati, and Bijoyama—who had finished their School Reading Certificate Course (graduation from high school) about the time Bela came to Mitraniketan. Bela invited the girls to work with her.

At the beginning their training was very elementary. "The first lesson was to clean the table," Suvarna remembered. "We learned that cleanliness is the first lesson of health."

Although sometimes in the evenings the health workers would sit for a formal class, which either Bela or Dr. Kohler would teach, much of the training took place on the job. "Sanitation, nutrition, hygiene—all the subjects were taught through practical work," Bijoyama told me.

The girls received clinic training by working closely with Bela when patients came for treatment. Home visits were also an important part of their training. Even after the health center was built, many women continued to have their babies delivered at home. For several days after each home delivery, Bela and the health workers made daily home visits to give the mothers suggestions for the baby's care. Bela used these occasions for informal instruction to the health workers.

To learn nutrition, the health workers helped in the kitchen. Bela taught them how to plan balanced meals for the Mitraniketan staff and the school hostel children. They assisted the cook with meal preparation and serving.

Under Bela's direction, the health workers brought the Mitraniketan kitchen expenses into line with the money allocated for the purpose. She taught the health workers to handle the accounts, to keep accurate records, to balance the books daily, and to plan economical purchases.

The health workers placed a high priority on their lessons in careful money management and the values they were taught in the process. When I asked Bijoyama what she learned from Bela that was most important to her, the answer came immediately. "Public health. And to be honest."

She explained: "I was only 17 years old, and I was not much acquainted with money. But she gave me the responsibility of the dining hall. She taught that each and every *paisa* (penny) should be correct and accounted for."

Bijoyama described the same kind of arrangement in accounting for the medicines in the clinic. She said that at Mitraniketan "no one ever took without telling." When she hears of workers stealing medicines from a clinic, she thinks of her health worker training. "We did not learn like that; Bela-chechi taught us not to do like that," she said.

Bela taught values by the example of her own life, but in addition, she had an unusual ability to verbalize her sense of values. She attributed her values to the influence of her mother and her half brother Satish. "If you do the right work and keep honest yourself, and are loving to the people, then you will be successful wherever you go. In my home these were the most important things we were taught," she told me.

"One thing I used to tell the health workers," Bela remembered, "was that when you are working you musn't think how much salary you are getting. You might not get anything and you might get a lot, but work and salary are not connected. They are different things. When you work sincerely, you will not think whether you are getting money or not. You shouldn't have that kind of mind."

At Mitraniketan, more than any other place where she worked, Bela was able to do what she envisioned in working with children. Even family planning was a concept that she considered important to instill in the minds of children. "I used to talk about big family and small family, how it is different," she told me. She talked to the children about the advantages of small families, pointing out that more education, food, and clothes can be provided for children in small families.

Frequently Bela used art as a teaching tool in the classes she taught at the Mitraniketan School. "I gave the children paper and crayons," she told me, "and I asked them to make me a picture of a house and a family in front of the house. I talked to them about the things the house should have. So they drew a picture of a house with a window, and a well, latrine, compost pit—we talked about these things and then they drew them. Then they drew a few flowers, trees in the back, and a kitchen garden beside the well. 'And then how many people should be in that house?' we asked, and they always said, 'Father, mother, and two children.' Or some said, 'three children.' Nobody said more than three. So always keeping in their mind two or three children would be enough, this is the way they grew up with the feeling of getting smaller families."

Suvarna, who now works at the government primary health center in her home village of Vellanad, described how Bela talked to the children in the health classes at the schools. "Very skillfully she could make little children understand about this small family idea. She would say, 'If your mother had only two bananas, and she had four children, how could you get one banana for yourself?' And the children could very easily say they would get only a small piece. 'But if there were only two, you could have one banana for each person,'" Subarna remembered Bela telling the children. "And gradually she could get across this idea and they knew it was better to have a smaller number than a big family of seven or eight children."

The Mitraniketan health workers whom I met talked about the outreach of the health classes into the homes. "In the health classes, we discussed using latrines and other health habits. Then the children talked about it with their parents. And every month we had parents' meetings, mothers' meetings, cooking classes, all arranged by Bela-chechi," said one of the health workers, using the Malayalam affectionate form of Bela's name as she talked about her. "At the parents' meetings and the mothers' meetings Bela would ask parents of children if they had latrines. People are more conscious now of the connection between sanitation and health," she concluded.

Three or four times a week Bela and her health workers taught classes at the Mitraniketan school. They also taught classes in two public schools and in a nearby mission school. Several of the later health workers had been Mitraniketan students who had known Bela through the health classes in the school.

After Dr. Kohler came to Mitraniketan she wrote to Dr. Morgan at Community Services about Bela's work: "All of Bela's efforts are very effective in the living patterns of the people here, and there is just no way of measuring all the things she has prevented and the miseries she has spared through her tireless teaching of public health precepts."

Because of her experiences at the AFSC project in Orissa, Bela provided impetus for the introduction of sanitary water-seal latrines in the Vellanad area. Several people told me about the latrine program at Mitraniketan. "Everybody came to look at the *kahcous* (latrines) that were made here," one woman said. "It was a big thing. Bela was very excited about it, and her enthusiasm spread to everybody else."

She laughed, remembering. "It became a status symbol, really. Everyone had to have their *kahcous*. Whenever we went visiting, instead of the first thing being to admire the baby, it was to come and look at the *kahcous*."

One year during the celebration of *Onam*, a religious holiday when young people in Kerala give presents to their parents, Saraswati and her husband gave a latrine to his parents in another village. Occasionally people bought a latrine because of its popularity, sometimes using the cement slab as a washboard to launder their clothing instead of its intended purpose. One of Bela's friends said she had teased someone who bought a latrine but did not install it: "Why don't you put some flowers in front of it and use it as a shrine; you have to do something with it."

When Caroline Balderston arrived to teach at the Mitraniketan school she asked the children in her first class to draw a picture for her, thinking that would be a good way to learn what some of their interests were. After class was over, she came running to Bela, laughing. "Bela, what have you taught the children? I asked them to draw a picture for me, and they all drew a picture of a latrine!"

Several workers told me about the health classes in the schools. "They were great fun. The children always enjoyed going," one person said.

Viswan attached great importance to Bela's teaching methods. He told me how she had borrowed a microscope so the children could see worms in stool specimens. "Then in their classes she asked them to draw pictures, and they have that consciousness—they draw pictures of the worms and of the *kahcous*," Viswan said. "That is the main thing, they will never forget about it. Now people in development talk about 'conscientization'—well, all that is done is to show that seeing is believing."

Sushila, one of the children in the Mitraniketan nursery school, was particularly active and serious in promoting the use of latrines. The path to the school from Sushila's home and several other homes around Vellanad went past the back of the health center. Sometimes on the way to or from school, one of the children would stop along the path to relieve himself and Sushila would take offense. "I will tell

Bela-chechi—you going outside, you not using the latrine," she would shout in a voice loud enough that Bela could hear her from the health center.

When Bela and I visited Mitraniketan, we stopped along the road next to Sushila's home. The house was a small, earthen building, the outer walls smoothed with cow-dung plaster, the dirt yard swept to a hard surface. Bela commented on its cleanliness. While we were standing beside the gate, Sushila's mother and sister recognized Bela and hurried out of the house to greet her.

"You have lost so much weight," Bela said to Sushila's mother. A man who had been walking along with us said, "Even after so many years she is concerned about our health."

Viswan spoke of the health education program in broad terms, citing Bela's contribution in maternal health and prevention of illness. He said she accomplished her goals through her visits to families to create awareness, and by working with school children in combining health classes with art. He described the outreach effect of Bela's health classes. "It was a pioneering work. And though we have not sought any publicity, many primary health center medical officers every year used to come here to see what was being done.

Roo Glazebrook remembered a nutrition project Bela undertook with the school children. "She was trying to get over the idea that eating doesn't mean you have to have rice all the time, that you can eat more vegetables. She introduced *chappaties*, (a whole wheat bread commonly eaten in north India but not known to many in Kerala). And again she had very good psychology in the way she did it." Roo described how Bela would plan the school dinner to include vegetables and *chappaties*. If the children liked the new food, they would go home and tell their parents and they would try it. "That way she got across her idea much better than if she had preached to them," Roo said.

Another part of Bela's nutrition education was to encourage people to grow vegetables, and she grew tomatoes and other vegetables herself. She also advised families to eat fruit. "It's much better to keep your bananas and give them to the children than to sell your bananas and buy biscuits," she told parents.

After two years of working with Suvarna, Saraswati, and Bijoyama, Bela expanded the health worker program to include others in the training. Shanta, our hostess during the 25th anniversary festivities at Mitraniketan, had been in the second group of young women to receive health worker training; she had begun her study with Bela after she graduated from high school in 1969.

When some of the health workers had a chance to get a government job or to take additional training to qualify them for work elsewhere, Bela encouraged them. "That's good, really," she told me. "They are very good nurses. They really take an interest in their work. I don't mind if they go to government jobs or get a better salary somewhere else, as long as they do good work."

Bela was loyal and protective towards the health workers, looking out for what she saw as their best interests. Roo Glazebrook described a confrontation that she remembered about the health workers' pay. "The health workers had been told there was a financial crisis—and there just wasn't the money and they weren't getting it. Bela was very upset. I think eventually she funded it from her own," Roo said.

When families of the health workers built new homes or enlarged their small houses, Bela contributed financially if they were having difficulty. Often she cooked extra food in her room to share with the health workers. On special holidays she bought khadi (homespun) saris and blouse material for each health worker. When she went to Calcutta on vacation, she brought gifts back to them. "I could help them that way," she said.

The health workers had all come from low-income families in the Vellanad area. One was a barber's daughter. One's father was a laundryman. Some were children of cultivators, others of day laborers.

Bela trained 12 health workers during the years she worked at Mitraniketan. Of the first three health worker graduates, Suvarna and Bijoyama are now officers in primary health centers, Suvarna in her home village of Vellanad and Bijoyama in another area of Kerala. They hold classes for mothers in prenatal clinics, give instruction to patients who come for treatment, and visit the homes of the people in the Community Development Block where they are assigned. Bijoyama spoke to me of Bela's influence in her work. "I don't know how I can express the value of public health that she taught. All the things that we teach other people and that we are still following, we learned from her."

Saraswati, the other health worker from the first group of Mitraniketan trainees, is a child development specialist who integrates health, nutrition, family planning services, and informal education for parents in a child development service connected with the Kerala School Welfare Board. After she started her new work, Saraswati wrote to Bela, "Every bit of what you taught me is now coming into use for me."

Several of the young women who took health worker training from Bela ranked first in their classes when they took nurses' training. When two of them got jobs at the Ramakrishna Mission Hospital in Trivandrum, the doctor there was very pleased about their work and told Bela, "They are very honest and sincere, and very good work they do."

Recognizing Bela's role in the high qualifications of the nurses, the doctor in charge of the hospital arranged for two groups of 12 Bachelor of Science nursing students from Kerala University to come to Mitraniketan to study with Bela for three months in rural health.

Sarama Thomas, one of Bela's health workers, had additional training and became a nurse practitioner in one of the Kasturba Gandhi Memorial Trust projects in northern Kerala.

Sharmala was a teenager delivering laundry for her father, the *dhobi* (washerman) for Mitraniketan, when she first met Bela and became a health worker trainee. After she worked with Bela for seven years, she was accepted for a leprosy health visitors program where she now works.

Another health worker and her husband organized an *ashram* (a social work center) to work with tribal people in the Kerala jungle.

A significant facet of Bela's work is the way in which she relates to individuals and spreads her ideas through individuals. "I'm sure that is why she is so successful—because she does start small," Roo Glazebrook said. "She started with three trainees—girls from three local families she met in the village."

Roo went on to generalize from the example. "I think that is where so many who try to help in India go wrong," she said. "You shouldn't leap in and pour in lots of money and lots of foreign people, and then leave after a year—which seems to be the general idea in western development projects. But you should actually work with the people that are there, starting on a personal basis. I think people will change if they see the point and purpose of it. And somebody with Bela's magnetism will attract people; they are very interested in her. They like her and therefore are prepared to listen to her."

Bela's acceptance in the community and the confidence people placed in her health workers led to success in her effort to combat local superstitions that affected people's health. One of these superstitions related to a belief that eating papaya caused miscarriages. Even though papaya was a common local fruit, easy to grow, inexpensive to buy, and a readily available source of Vitamin A in the diet, pregnant women did not eat the fruit.

Bela began a campaign to prove the superstition wrong. She distributed papaya plants from the Mitraniketan garden to every home she visited. She emphasized the importance of a nutritious diet when she talked to the women receiving prenatal care. She included papaya in the list of healthful foods to eat during pregnancy.

Even then, not many women were willing to eat papaya if they were pregnant, until Saraswati, one of Bela's health workers, became pregnant and Bela gave her papaya to eat. Saraswati's trust in Bela overcame her hesitancy to eat the fruit. As other pregnant women watched Saraswati's successful pregnancy and ultimate delivery of a healthy full-term baby, they too began to discard the superstition.

Bela's health workers were not only trained to do routine work, but they learned to cope with emergencies as well. Joan Evison, a young British woman who visited Mitraniketan in 1968, had been at the project for less than a week when she had an accident that badly scalded a large part of her body. After giving first aid Bela organized transport for Joan to the nearest hospital in Trivandrum, an hour's drive across mountainous terrain, over what seemed to Joan to be unmade roads and tracks.

Although the hospital at Trivandrum was a good one, providing the medical care she needed, Joan found the system strange and frightening, because the nonmedical care of patients was not the responsibility of the hospital staff but of the patients' families. Fulfilling the function of family, Bela and the Mitraniketan health workers stayed with Joan in shifts, so that someone was always with her. Even though the health workers had learned only a little English so that communication with Joan was mostly by smiles except when Bela was there, Joan was comforted by the health workers' constant presence. Each day the shift changed, as the health workers traded back and forth to spend time with Joan, traveling a half day by bus by the time they reached the hospital from Mitraniketan. For some of them, it may have been their first time outside their village area, the first time they had traveled on a bus or been to Trivandrum. "That they did this—and were able to do it—was basically Bela's achievement, unheard of and unrecorded, happening in a remote corner of India," Joan wrote, telling about the experience.

One of the programs that Bela organized at Mitraniketan involved weekly visits to provide medical care and food to people who lived in three tribal colonies in the mountains not far from Vellanad. Roo Glazebrook, who often went with Bela and the health workers, described the situation. "We would drive the jeep into the jungle; it would seem as though there was nobody around. Then we would stop the jeep and blow the horn. For a moment nothing would happen. Then suddenly people began appearing, coming out from the forest into the clearing."

Many of the tribal people suffered from malnutrition. Trying to alleviate the extreme malnutrition among children in the colonies, Bela and the health workers cooked food at Mitraniketan to distribute to the children, along with CARE food packages. "It was difficult to decide which of the many children needed it most," Bela said.

Bela and the health workers also visited the tribal people in their homes, talking to them about hygiene. Eventually Bela invited a girl from each of the three colonies to come to Mitraniketan for health worker training. When their training was finished they went back to the colonies to serve as health workers.

At the close of Mitraniketan's silver anniversary celebration, Viswanathan visited with me about Bela's influence. He started by citing recent accomplishments in the community that had come about because of Bela's earlier work. The Vellanad primary school had won a national health award, primarily, Viswan believes, because they adopted the health program Bela had initiated years before. He described the neat, clean school surroundings. He said that the school latrines installed because of Bela's health classes were still used and maintained. The garden that was started at her suggestion continued to produce vegetables for the school children's meals.

Viswan switched in his thinking from school children to their mothers and other adults, as he spoke of Bela's influence in the Vellanad area. "Bela's life is a message to the women, particularly young women," he said. "She is a self-made woman. She has built herself up through her own effort. And, of course, she has hosts of friends. You cannot simply get friends unless you have that friendliness within you, and the love that has just overflowed from the friendship. Bela's work is all practical experience. Social work, nursing. I wish there would be more people just hearing and drawing inspiration from such life patterns. She has a message to the world."

Viswan continued, comparing Bela to Mother Theresa in Calcutta. "I don't think that Bela's work is in any way inferior to the work of Mother Theresa. Consider Beladi's life and the work she has done—she has put in many, many years of service, and it is behind the curtain only. Nobody was there to lift the curtain as there was when Mother Theresa was made known to the whole world. There are no big organizations or forces behind Bela, except her good friends; that is the difference between Mother Theresa and her.

"The persons who had the opportunity to know Bela and her work, they all have a lot of praise," Viswan went on. "We have used her—her good will, her talents—but we also have a moral obligation . . . we should let the world know, particularly in India. People can build up confidence, courage, the passion to know things, to do things through knowing her story. We need hundreds of thousands of Beladis."

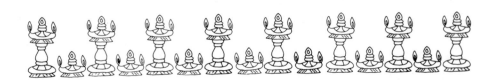

20
HEALTH CARE AT FRIENDS RURAL CENTRE

Our trip from Kerala to our destination in Madhya Pradesh was the longest segment of the journey that Bela Banerjee and I made together. The first train took us back to Madras where we had a lay-over of several hours, as we had done on the way down from Bhubaneswar.

As we rode along, we had a good view of the Kerala countryside—the vivid colors of the sun on backwater bays, houses thatched with palm branches, sometimes the walls constructed of the same material woven into mats, fields of tapioca plants interspersed with banana trees and coconut palms, women transplanting rice from seedbeds into rows in the fields, water buffalo bathing in the village ponds, and children waving at the train.

At the Trivandrum station an elderly woman in a heavy cotton village *sari* had approached us, traveling alone and wanting companionship on the train. We compared tickets and when she saw that she was assigned to a different coach than we were, she went on. Bela said, "I know just how she feels. I usually travel alone, and I never like it." When we reached Madras, we saw the woman again, and she smiled broadly, as if to say, "I made it this far."

At Madras we transferred to an express train to travel the long journey—about 30 hours—to Itarsi. The transition from the southern part of the country to central India was accompanied by changes in the cries of the vendors who sold their wares through the train windows at each station stop. "Coffee-loffee-offee. Nes-coffee. Bru-coffee. Coffee-loffee-offee," was the rapid, melodious call that prompted us to purchase a cup of coffee in the south. (Although their sales pitch named two different brands, the coffee—already sweetened and lightened with milk—was always poured from a single kettle.) As we traveled north, the call that penetrated the night air and blended into other early morning sounds was more frequently a slow chant at a single lower voice pitch, advertising *"chai, garam chai* (tea, hot tea)." During the daytime Bela and I had long conversations, punctuated with the rhythm of the train wheels clicking along the rails and occasional loud whistles as the engine pulled into stations.

From Itarsi we rode for an hour on a crowded bus to reach the Friends Rural Centre in the village of Rasulia, where Bela had worked for a year beginning in January 1974.

Friends Rural Centre has a long history, having been started by British Quakers about 1888 as an industrial training school for orphan boys. After 30 years the school was closed, but in 1934 British and Indian Quakers reopened the center to begin a community development project that was closely correlated with Gandhian methods of village development. In the 1950s the project took on characteristics of the post-war western development model, becoming a sister project of Barpali Village Service when the American Friends Service Committee joined with the British Friends Service Council to co-sponsor both projects.

Focusing first on education and later on agriculture, Friends Rural Centre made only minimal efforts to provide a health program until the late 1950s. At that time, a few years after their term at Barpali Village Service had ended, Edwin and Vivien Abbott returned to India to work at the Rasulia project. As they had done at Barpali, the Abbotts began a clinic and a public health program that concentrated on pump wells and latrines as effective means to prevent disease.

Bela had visited Friends Rural Centre several times while the Abbotts were at the project, but they had returned to their home in Canada before she went there to work. When the Australian nurse and British doctor who had replaced the Abbotts were finishing their terms, Friends Rural Centre invited Bela to work in the health education program. Bela, requesting a year's leave from Mitraniketan, saw the Rasulia appointment as an opportunity to think through her future plans.

Bela felt a close rapport with Ashoke Chopra, the Punjabi doctor with whom she worked at Friends Rural Centre. Especially in the public health program, Dr. Chopra looked to Bela for leadership. "He listened to what I said," she told me. "He and I always used to have a conference and talk about the work we were doing."

Bela described how Dr. Chopra dealt with patients. "The village people always liked to have their pulse taken, so he used to sit there, holding the patient's wrist and asking how is the man's wife, how many children, how much land, house condition—all these things he used to ask, instead of only saying, "What is wrong with you?" That impressed me so much," she added.

The patients responded to the doctor's approach. "All the patients liked him," Bela remembered. "I was really fond of him, because of this one reason—he was so good to the patients, and I thought right away that he was really a good doctor."

The medical team with whom Bela worked at Friends Rural Centre was small. In addition to Dr. Chopra and Bela there was Sita Kapur, a part-time nurse who worked with family planning patients; two health workers, Kamala and Sushila; and Santosh, a young man who gave medication to tuberculosis patients. During the year at Rasulia, Bela trained another health worker—also named Sushila—a young woman from Rasulia whom she met on one of her visits to village homes.

The clinic at Friends Rural Centre included general health care, prenatal care, and postnatal care, but not deliveries of babies. Except that she did not include midwifery training, Bela trained Sushila in the same informal way she had conducted the classes at Mitraniketan. The Rasulia routine included morning clinics and home visits in the afternoons. In the home visits Bela and the health workers told people about the clinic and provided health education in the homes. Their pattern was to visit each house once, and then to return wherever they were invited.

Bela attempted to change some of the beliefs that many people around Rasulia held regarding pregnancy and childbirth. They believed, for example, that pregnant women shouldn't eat tomatoes. When they learned to trust Bela, however, some of them became convinced that tomatoes were safe to eat.

Because childbirth was considered to be unclean, traditionally no attempt was made to maintain a sterile environment during delivery. The midwife was another village woman, sometimes an aunt or other relative and sometimes a woman from a particular caste of midwives. Sometimes the village midwives used broken pieces of earthen pot to cut the cord; other times they used razor blades, but without sterilization.

To counteract these practices, Bela showed the women a picture of someone cutting the cord with dirty broken pottery, juxtaposed with a picture of a baby with tetanus. Another set of pictures showed cleanliness during delivery—the midwife washing her hands with soap, boiling scissors, and providing clean cloths; it was associated with a picture of a healthy baby.

Although Bela had been given a one-year leave from Mitraniketan, she might have continued her term at Rasulia for a longer time, except that Dr. Chopra decided to leave the project. After he left, the project coordinator asked Bela, "Do you want to stay or do you want to go?" Because the new doctor did not work as a team with Bela and the health workers and was not interested in the health education program, Bela decided to return to Mitraniketan.

In viewing the various areas of the work at Friends Rural Centre, Bela noticed other changes in the project direction. While she was at Rasulia, for example, the coordinator of the project cut down all the orange, lemon and lime trees in the orchard and planted new varieties of fruit, a move she considered "too extreme." In her contact with the project, Bela noted a change of policy with each change of leadership. Speaking of the different administrators, she said, "Each one had his own ideas what was right."

Bela's personal approach to development was, as she said, "to keep it level." Changes in direction that were unrelated to the villagers' own understanding of their needs did not correspond to Bela's methods of identifying closely with the people among whom she worked.

Marjorie Sykes, a long-time adviser to both of the Quaker projects in India, was hostess at the Friends Rural Centre at the time of our visit. Through the years since they have become friends, Bela has looked to Marjorie frequently for guidance in her vocational plans. Her year in Rasulia had been at Marjorie's suggestion, and when Bela and I arrived for our brief visit, they eagerly renewed their friendship.

At Friends Rural Centre in 1982, Partap Aggarwal, the new coordinator, had redirected the agricultural focus of the project to emphasize environmental concerns related to farming. Bela did not understand the implications of the change of focus, and she was concerned that a relationship be maintained with the local farmers. She saw involvement with the people as the vital element of development. "I think the people are more important than just the land and doing the work to grow lots of food," she said.

Bela was pleased with the morning meeting of all the project workers that Aggarwal had started. The meeting each day began with a reading and discussion of the Gandhian leader Vinoba Bhave's writings about the *Bhagavad Gita*, the Hindu scriptures. Then the workers talked about the day's work and any problems they had encountered the day before. They discussed directions they wanted to go and exchanged advice with one another. Everyone from the grass cutters that fed the cattle in the dairy to the project coordinator was expected to attend, and most of them did. The atmosphere at the meeting was one of camaraderie with a great deal of interchange of ideas. The morning we were there, a group of students had come from an agricultural college to look at the methane gas plant at the center, and they began their day at the morning meeting also.

At the time of our visit to Rasulia the clinic was virtually closed, with only an occasional illness of the Friends Rural Centre workers being treated. Santosh continued to provide medication to tuberculosis patients when they came to him, but few did. Bela was disappointed that the medical program had diminished.

Two medical problems occurred during our visit to the Friends Rural Centre, and Bela was called upon to deal with both. One of the emergencies happened when another Rasulia guest fell and injured her shoulder while she was trying to adjust the mosquito netting over her bed. Bela looked at the injury and decided that she should take the woman to the hospital in a nearby town to have her shoulder x-rayed. After waiting all afternoon, they were told that the x-ray could not be done there, so Partap took the woman to a private doctor where it was discovered that she had chipped a bone.

In the evening Bela and I visited with Marjorie Sykes while she was cooking. Bela told us about the conditions at the hospital where they had spent the afternoon. "I would like to go to that hospital and just do cleaning, because it smelled so bad," she said. Marjorie and I laughed, and Bela said, "Really, I feel that way—that sometime I should just come there and do nothing except just clean away."

We were still visiting with Marjorie when Partap came to get Bela to look at a sick child of one of the workers in the compound. The child had been sick with a fever all day and was having a convulsion when they called for Bela. Bela looked at the child and advised his parents to try to bring the fever down with ice. Later the child had another convulsion and Bela was called again. When no one could locate the clinic equipment she needed, Bela advised the child's parents to take him to the hospital. By then Partap was gone with the project jeep. The parents decided to carry the child on a bicycle and walk alongside. Just then someone drove into the project compound on a motorcycle and agreed to take the child to the hospital. The father rode along to carry the little boy. As Partap was returning with the jeep he met the child's mother who had starting walking the three miles to the hospital; he gave her a ride to the hospital and then brought the family back to the project after the child was treated by a doctor.

Only a few of Bela's co-workers were still at Friends Rural Centre. One of them who had remained was Subatra Misra, whose husband Jagdeesh was the project accountant. Subatra called Bela her sister when she greeted her. She was concerned that Bela "looked tired, so thin."

Subatra had been Bela's neighbor at the project, and they had developed a close friendship. "If Bela didn't come to my house, I would go to hers," Subatra said.

Bela said, "She used to bring food to me."

"Oh, yes. That was nothing," Subatra said.

"And she gave me a *sari* from Calcutta that I still wear," Bela said.

Jagdeesh Misra said, "She is like our own family in her relationship with us."

During our visit to Friends Rural Centre, Bela washed a *sari* and asked Subatra if she could hang it on the line on her verandah. Giving her consent, Subatra said, "You shouldn't ask; this is your sister's house."

Subatra talked to me about Bela's work at Friends Rural Centre, her husband interpreting her Hindi into English. "When she was at Rasulia, she was like mother, sister, everything to us," Subatra said. "She used to get up anytime anybody was sick; she would come and see and look after everybody. She is more than a doctor. Many good doctors were here; Bela was just like one of them. Bela used to go to the village to take care of babies and children," Subatra said. "Old people, village people—they all think about her."

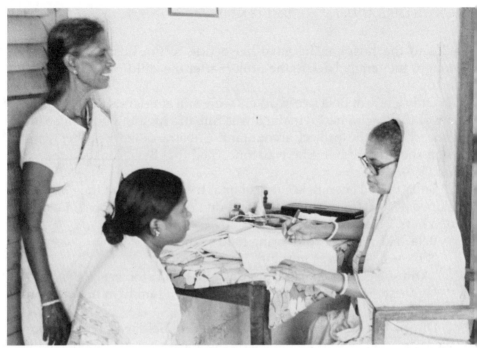

Bela with Dr. Tungavidya and a health worker in the clinic at the Orissa head-quarters of the Kasturba Gandhi National Memorial Trust, Satyabhamapur, 1982.

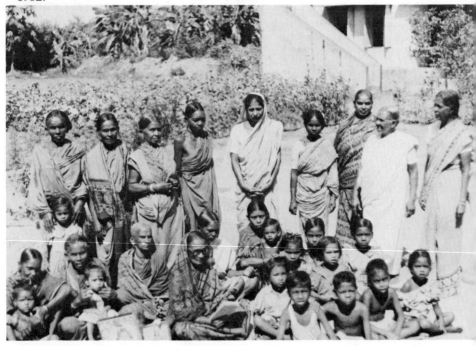

Members of the women's group, the nursery, and the staff at the Dhama-Bargaon KGNMT center meeting with Bela, 1982.

PART SEVEN:

ORISSA: WORK WITH CHILDREN

"Let me light my lamp,"
    says the star,
        "And never debate
if it will help to remove the darkness."

—Rabindranath Tagore
from *Fireflies*

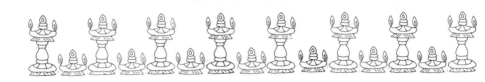

21
AT HOME IN MANY HOMES

During the year Bela worked at Rasulia, Olive Grabham, her closest friend from her nurses training years at Royal Free Hospital, came to India to visit her for three months. Bela went to Calcutta to meet Olive and the two of them stayed a few days with Bela's family and friends there before going back to Rasulia and then to Mitraniketan and Barpali so that Olive could see where Bela had worked since completing her nurses' training.

While she was visiting at Rasulia, Olive Grabham gave Bela money for a plane ticket to England, but by the time Bela's passport was issued, the plane fare had gone up, so that she no longer had enough money to buy the ticket. By then, she had returned to Mitraniketan. At first she thought she would have to give up the idea for the trip and decided to remain at Mitraniketan until other possibilities for work seemed right to her.

Early in 1976, Bela wrote to her friend Eleanor Eaton about a job possibility in Calcutta. A friend in Calcutta had offered her a house near the Dum Dum airport where she could begin a health center for needy children and their mothers. Bela envisioned the project as being patterned after the Friends Centre on Upper Wood Street, where she had first become associated with Quakers. Marjorie Sykes visited the house with Bela and was willing to back her in the project. Some other friends helped her plan a budget, and she wrote to Eleanor Eaton to see if friends in the United States might provide financial support.

Before the plan materialized, however, the house that she had hoped to use for a maternal and child health center was sold. Nonetheless, Bela still had the dream. Later in the year, she decided to leave Mitraniketan even though she had no firm plans for the future; she returned to Calcutta and stayed with her friends Sati and Bhupen Ghose while she explored various possibilities for employment. Thinking of the many schools in Kerala where the health workers she had trained in Mitraniketan were invited to teach health classes, she began to consider the possibility of starting a center for health workers to receive training to teach public health in lower primary schools so that children could grow up with better health habits. But she did not know how to implement the idea.

She looked at a possible job in an institution for emotionally disturbed children in Calcutta, but that work also did not materialize.

Bela's friends offered other suggestions. Marjorie Sykes encouraged her to return to Rasulia to train health workers, or to do similar work in a project in the Nilgiri Hills of South India. Those jobs would take her farther away from her family and friends, but not so far as Mitraniketan. Indubhushan Misra suggested that she work with a young doctor in a backward village in eastern Orissa, within a day's journey of Calcutta. None of the ideas developed into work opportunities for her.

Finally Bela learned of another project in Orissa that seemed to give her a possible new direction. One of her Barpali Village Service health workers had established three centers for orphans, following a famine in the state in 1975. She invited Bela to manage one of the centers. For four months Bela lived there, camping out in a temporary earthen shed. While she was there she worked with government officials to get grants for housing and to provide better food and medical care for the children. She talked to British Oxfam workers to obtain a pump well for drinking water. By the time the monsoon rains began, no building had been started for workers' housing, and Bela had been ill with malaria and dysentery several times. She decided that she should not continue at the center.

By then Olive Grabham realized that the money she had given was no longer sufficient to cover the cost of a plane ticket to London and she sent Bela the remainder that was needed. The timing seemed right for Bela to go to England and she postponed the decision about her future work.

In July 1977 the arrangements were completed and she made the trip, landing at the London airport with scarcely any money because she was not allowed to take *rupees* out of India. She telephoned her nephew Samiran and he came to London from his home in Chelmsford, Essex, to meet her at the airport. She stayed with Samiran and Parboti and their three daughters for a couple of weeks. "When she came here she just wouldn't sit down," Parboti told me when I visited her and Samiran in England. Bela had noticed that Samiran had a garden where he grew vegetables, and she at once took over the cooking, preparing the food the way she knew from her childhood that he enjoyed. "She's a wonderful cook," Parboti said, and Lela, one of her daughters agreed, and told me about the coconut pancakes that Bela had cooked for her. Parboti described Bela as "both an indoor and an outdoor person," combining domestic qualities with a career and travel.

After her visit with Samiran's family, Bela went to Cambridge to see Joan Court and then to Folkestone in Kent to be with Olive Grabham. When Bela came, Olive's 92-year old mother was seriously ill. Bela had become close friends with Olive's mother when she and Olive were nursing students and again on her trip in 1963. Now she was distressed that she had not been able to visit Olive's mother again before the elderly woman became extremely ill. "We hoped my mother knew it was Bela, because she had looked forward so to seeing her," Olive said.

So that neither Samiran nor Olive would need to be responsible for her expenses, Bela set out to find work for the six months she planned to be in England.

At the time of Bela's arrival, Joan Court had just moved to Cambridge where she was enrolled in a social work doctoral program. She arranged for Bela to stay in the house where she had been living in London, where Bela could earn money as a companion to the owner of the house, a 90-year old woman named Miss St. Barbe.

According to Hetty Budgen, who visited Bela at Miss St. Barbe's house, "Bela fitted beautifully into the house and did everything for Miss St. Barbe while she was there." Bela had a quality of "gentleness and an instinctive way that she could look after people," Hetty Budgen said. "And she loved looking after people, so she just took Miss St. Barbe under her wing."

Miss St. Barbe had been in the habit of wandering away from home. She would insist on going shopping and then would become completely lost. People in the area who knew her would bring her back home. With Bela there to keep an eye on her, to cook for her and to be a companion to her, Miss St. Barbe's life was more secure and, according to Hetty Budgen, Miss St. Barbe "absolutely adored Bela."

For Bela the trip to England was a time to meet old friends and also a time for observing various projects and institutions to get ideas of work she might want to do when she returned to India. Joan Court arranged for many of these study tours, so that Bela could observe various social work projects for children, foster care facilities, day care centers for physically handicapped, and other kinds of community work relating to families.

On this visit, Margot Tennyson recognized Bela's feelings of uncertainty about her future. "Bela always was someone of tremendous courage," Margot said. "She had very little security, and she had a desire to be useful, but she made this trip without knowing what she was going back to. She has been very plucky."

With a six-month visa to England and a return airline ticket good for a year, Bela began to lay plans for a side trip to the United States. She wrote to friends at the American Friends Service Committee offices in Philadelphia. Eleanor Eaton and Robert Gray—both of them former directors at Barpali Village Service—set up the plans. Contacting Bela's friends in North America, Eleanor and Robert raised money for her airline ticket to the United States and for a bus ticket in the states.

She traveled as far west as Kansas and Nebraska, visiting friends along the way. From Michigan, where she stayed in the home of David and Miyoko Bassett, doctors who had worked with her at the Barpali project, she flew back to the east coast. On almost all her previous long distance traveling Bela had been alone, but the flight from Ann Arbor to Philadelphia stands out in her memory because Miyoko Bassett was with her on the trip. "It was the best travel of my life, really," Bela said, describing her enjoyment of Miyoko's companionship on the flight.

Early in 1978 Bela flew back to England for several weeks, where she continued to visit social work centers and hospitals. "It was interesting to see what they do in homes to help handicapped people, children and old people," she wrote to a friend in the United States.

Side trips to the Netherlands and to France completed Bela's trip, and she returned to India in April. Soon afterwards she wrote to friends she had visited on her trip, "I look forward to my dream become true—making a home in India where I will be welcoming you all and you may feel as much at home as you made me feel during my stay [in your homes]."

Bela had accepted a job at the *Seva Samiti,* a project for women and children near the Orissa village of Haridaspur. Indubhushan Misra had made the arrangements for her to take the position, while she was still on her trip to England and the United States. She had been staying with Eleanor Eaton in New Jersey when she received Indu's letter, asking if she wanted to work there, and Eleanor had written to him on her behalf, encouraging him to complete the plans.

"I felt that in India, Indu is the person who will always help me. When he found this place, everybody was pleased about it," Bela said. "If it was Indu's suggestion it must be a good place, Eleanor and the other friends in the U.S. thought."

Indu was acquainted with the project at Haridaspur and knew Rhombadevi, the founder. As a government supervisor of schools he had established a primary school which the *Seva Samiti* operated along with a nursery school. The main work of the *Seva Samiti* centered around a hospital with 35 beds and intensive maternity care in neighboring villages.

Nityananda Patnaik, an anthropologist who had been a rural life analyst at Barpali Village Service and who was then in charge of the Orissa Government Tribal Welfare Department, was also interested in Rhombadevi's project because it provided services to tribal people who lived in the area. Nitu's wife Ranga had been one of Bela's health workers at BVS; she had worked closely with Kamala Misra when their husbands had been technicians at the Barpali project.

Eager to help Bela become situated in her new work, the Misras and Patnaiks accompanied her on the train. When they reached Haridaspur an hour later than the scheduled 10:00 p.m. arrival time, no one was there to meet them. Not knowing where to spend the night in the village, Bela and her four friends walked the two to three kilometers into the hilly scrub jungle to reach the *Seva Samiti*.

Bela generally traveled light, with only a suitcase even on her longest trips. This time, however, since she was going to be living at the *Seva Samiti*, she had more baggage than usual. Indu and Nitu took the heaviest luggage, both of them lifting it to their heads in the style of Indian coolies, and started down the path. Bela laughed, making a play on words, "Head of anthropology and head of education are carrying my luggage on their heads."

Bela knew that the director Rhombadevi was dedicated to improving the lives of the villagers in the area. Nonetheless, as she became acquainted at Haridaspur, she saw serious gaps in the content of the program. Very poor sanitation and the lack of any agricultural program affected the nutrition and health conditions in the villages.

Neither milk nor fruit was available for the children in the nursery school or for patients in the hospital.

Bela described the *Seva Samiti* in a letter she wrote to Eleanor Eaton shortly after her arrival at Haridaspur. "Main work is hospital. Also outdoor clinic and village work. There are almost 200 small children in the nursery school." She continued, telling about the low standards of public health she had noticed. "When I see that, I feel bad. No nutrition program, no vegetable growing, although water and places are enough (for growing gardens), no latrine, except a few for use by project staff. No health education. Hospital is very dirty."

As usual, Bela had a plan to change the conditions. "I want to do public health work, take classes to the children and the workers, organize vegetable growing and latrine-making program," she wrote to Eleanor.

Bela offered classes to the hospital staff, but there were too few staff members to do the hospital work in order to free others to take the classes.

For a short while Bela taught classes in personal hygiene, sanitation, nutrition, and family planning in the Haridaspur School. Once she held a camp for 45 village women for two weeks. The women were supposed to be National Extension Service Block village leaders in the areas of nutrition, sanitation, and family planning, but Bela found that they knew nothing of the subject matter, so she developed elementary class instruction for them in the three subjects.

Bela looked forward to the project's plan for a hostel for tribal girls. With the girls at the hostel she thought she could start a health worker training program. She also had hoped to get financial support for a dairy and agricultural program, but she did not find funds for either project.

Bela's pattern of working directly with her village neighbors was not practical in the Haridaspur area. Most of the 35 villages that were home to the patients at the hospital and the children at the school were too far for frequent visits on foot, and gas was too expensive to keep the project jeep running most of the time.

Perhaps part of Bela's frustration came because she could see similarities to Barpali, and yet she found no way to begin programs such as the AFSC project had undertaken. Across the top of an airletter to Eleanor Eaton she had written, "This place is so much like Barpali. It makes me sad that you are not with me."

Bela felt uncomfortable at Haridaspur, since she was not really able to do the sort of health education work that she had expected to do. Nonetheless, she was grateful to be in Orissa instead of Kerala, since it was possible to visit her family in West Bengal more frequently.

During the hot season in March 1979, Joan Bocock came to India to visit Bela and to see the place where she was working. Joan had been the principal sister tutor at the Royal Free Hospital in London when Bela was there for nurses' training. Bela went to Calcutta to meet Joan and took her to Haridaspur. It was gratifying to Joan Bocock to visit some of the places where Bela had worked after receiving her nurses' training under Joan's tutelage and to meet Bela's friends in West Bengal and Orissa.

To all of her friends in England and the United States, Bela extended frequent invitations to visit her in India. When one friend expressed a hope of coming to India, Bela did not let her forget. "I am very much waiting to see you [at the] end of this year; hope you have not forgotten that. I am very much excited for that day to arrive. Where and when you will be arriving, please let me know [and] I will meet you at the airport. I am very [eager] to show you around."

After each of her trips outside India, she continued to reminisce about the visits with her friends. While she was at Haridaspur, she wrote to Eleanor Eaton, "Often I see leaves from your yard which I collected when I was there. I put them in my notebook; it was beautiful color then."

Although Bela did not write frequent lettters to most of her friends, if she knew that a friend was ill, she wrote immediately and often. When she heard of a friend's death, she not only wrote at once to his wife, but took it upon herself to notify others in India who knew him also.

When babies were born to her friends, she designated an Indian name whose meaning was her wish for the child. "Ashish, which means blessing, is the Indian name I give your son," she wrote in response to one birth announcement that she received from a friend.

During most of the time Bela worked at Haridaspur, she suffered from a severe pain in her right arm. It had started almost at once after she returned home from her trip; one doctor diagnosed it as osteoporosis. She received what she described as "lots of treatment but not much improvement."

In August she wrote to a friend, "My right arm is very painful and I cannot do any heavy work. I have more pain in the night, so I feel very much worried. Doctor said it will go slowly and I shouldn't worry, but I have to depend on others to do so many things to do for me, which I do not like. People are here very nice to me, so I am well looked after. Otherwise I am fine and trying to do what I can."

During the year that Bela was at Haridaspur, Rhombadevi was serving as *pratinidhi* (director) of the Orissa Kasturba Gandhi National Memorial Trust, as well as managing the project at Haridaspur. When Rhombadevi became aware of Bela's interest in undertaking some more meaningful work than what was available to her at Haridaspur, she suggested that Bela be named *pratinidhi* in her place and move to Satyabhamapur where the Orissa headquarters were located.

Bela had never been an administrator, and her first reaction was that she would not be qualified to do the job. "I thought it is not possible for me because I don't know how to do the administrative work," she said. When she expessed her concern to Golak Das, the accountant for the Kasturba Trust, he offered to continue to take the lead in the administration of the trust, as he had been doing since the beginning of the Orissa projects. When Ramadevi Chaudhuri who had been the first *pratinidhi* and her daughter-in-law who had held the position for 14 years joined Rhombadevi in the invitation, Bela agreed to try it out. "They all together asked me to come and stay there, and they said they would all help me," she said. And so began another chapter in her life of service.

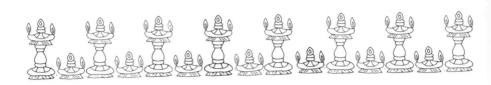

22
KASTURBA GANDHI
NATIONAL MEMORIAL TRUST

It was scarcely dawn on an October morning in 1982 when Bela and I left Misra's house in Bhubaneswar to make the journey to the village of Satyabhamapur where Bela was then working with the Kasturba Gandhi National Memorial Trust (KGNMT). Indubhushan Misra had gone out before us to find the driver of a bicycle rickshaw to take us and our overnight luggage—Bela's in a basket with a handle and mine in an over-the-shoulder tote bag—to the bus station.

Forty-five minutes after leaving Bhubaneswar, we changed buses in Cuttack. By 9:00 a.m. we were ten miles out of Cuttack, having reached Pagha, the village along the main road that is closest to Satyabhamapur. From there we went the final two and one-half miles to the KGNMT center by bicycle rickshaw. All the cycle rickshaw drivers waiting at the bus stop seemed to be Bela's friends. She laughed and joked with them and chose one to take us to Satyabhamapur.

A small jungle area divides the KGNMT compound. Linked by a narrow path, the two parts of the compound are fairly near one another, but if one stays on the road, as Bela and I did, the journey from the office, nursery school, and training school to the rest of the project is probably half a mile or so farther. Staying in the rickshaw, Bela and I rode into Satyabhamapur, turned a corner in the center of the small village, and a few yards down the road turned again so that we were headed back in the direction we had just come. From the village road we turned into a lane that led to the part of the center where Bela's room, the clinic, and the kitchen were located. These buildings formed three sides of a square surrounding an inner courtyard at the Kasturba project.

All the buildings were of cement or brick with clay tile roofs, except the kitchen which was made of earthen bricks and had a thatched roof. Folk paintings decorated the walls of the kitchen verandah. Behind the kitchen was the orphanage, a garden, and an orchard. In a small park outside Bela's front verandah were two small statues, busts of Mahatma Gandhi and of Modhu Shudan Das, the man who had previously owned the property where the Orissa Kasturba Trust headquarters are located.

The Kasturba Gandhi National Memorial Trust was started by Gandhi in 1945, a year after his wife's death. Each state of India collected contributions to the trust fund to support projects designed to benefit the poorest women and children of India. As the Orissa *pratinidhi* Bela was responsible for the administration of the ten projects in the state.

Ramadevi Chaudhuri, the first *pratinidhi* in Orissa, still maintained an interest in the KGNMT and was instrumental in getting Bela to accept the position. Bela was pleased to be associated with Ramadevi Chaudhury, a woman in her eighties, who had been a Gandhian social service worker all her adult life. "She has done wonderful work. I am glad I am with her," Bela said.

The feeling appeared to be mutual. When Ramadevi saw Laksmi Menon, chairman of the All-India KGNMT, who was also on the board of Mitraniketan where Bela had worked before returning to Orissa, she said to her, "You gave us a diamond." Laksmi Menon retorted with a smile. "You stole my diamond."

Bela went to the Satyabhamapur project in October 1979 and became *pratinidhi* the following April. She worked closely with Golak Chandra Das, the KGNMT accountant, whose efficient administrative leadership was invaluable to her. "We do it together—everything," Bela said. "When we go to government places to get grants, permits, find out about government regulations, I take him also."

The work of the Kasturba Trust is well recognized in Orissa. A documentary film was made about Ramadevi when she received an award for being a "great social worker." For more than two months Bela had accompanied the film crew to the Orissa KGNMT projects, and was in the film, both at Satyabhamapur and at a project in Koraput District.

When Bela and I arrived at the KGNMT center, everyone on the staff and the children in the orphanage came to meet us. Some of the girls bent over to touch Bela's feet in a formal greeting. Obviously uncomfortable with the show of reverence, Bela hurriedly urged them to stand up and then introduced me to the girls and to her co-workers.

Later in the day Bela and I toured the compound. Several girls from the orphanage were doing their laundry in the pond just in front of Bela's house and the clinic building. At the nursery school the children, obviously well-rehearsed for our arrival, shouted a greeting. "*Jai Jogot* (Victory to the world)!"

As Bela and I walked through the village, she stopped to talk with nearly everyone we met. A rickshaw driver sitting beside his empty cycle rickshaw questioned why we hadn't come earlier. She greeted a man sitting on a cot on his verandah, one leg in a cast, and told me he had broken his leg when he fell while thatching his roof.

In the evening everyone from the center gathered in the courtyard, where the girls from the orphanage sang and danced, accompanied by drums and a harmonium. Seven of the older girls, accomplished dancers, performed a *sari* dance, creating the images of a butterfly, a peacock, and a lotus flower. The tiny children sang an action song, and one very small girl sang a solo. Bela praised each presentation.

Afterwards Bela and I ate our dinner with other staff members, sitting on the floor and eating the vegetarian food in the Indian fashion without utensils.

Morning begins early at Gandhian centers. The prayer bell awakened us at 4:00 a.m., and soon afterwards we made our way to a large room where the girls from the orphanage were already seated on individual mats in rows facing the project staff. Two empty places on mats beside the doctor, on the front row of the area where the staff sat, had been designated for Bela and me. We sat down and the prayers began.

After an opening chant of "*shanti, shanti, shanti*, (peace, peace, peace,)" the other prayers were sung, some by two older girls who led the service and others by all the children and some of the staff. After prayers the girls stayed in the same room to practice yoga exercises, starting with the familiar "greeting to the sun." Appropriately, dawn was just then lightening the sky.

During the day I learned more about the work of the Satyabhamapur center. Besides serving as the Orissa headquarters for the Trust, the project operates an orphanage for 30 girls, a nursery school, an eight-bed hospital, an outpatient clinic, a health worker training program and a training program to increase employment possibilities for destitute women.

When Bela came to Satyabhamapur there was no doctor; three midwives handled about 130 delivery cases in the first six months Bela was there. Bela assisted with difficult cases, sometimes staying all night with women in labor.

Tungavidya-devi, who came to Satyabhamapur in 1981 had been the physician with the KGNMT at another project in Orissa for several years prior to her marriage in 1958. When she visited the Kasturba Trust projects after Bela had become *pratinidhi*, Bela invited her to return to establish a training program at the maternity center. She is the only doctor working with the Orissa KGNMT.

At Bela's suggestion Dr. Tungavidya began to train health workers in a ten-month program of hygiene, math, child care and spinning. Following the training, the young women agree to work for two years in the Maternity Center. An auxiliary nurse-midwife training program at the national Trust headquarters at Kasturbagram in Indore in western India provides an additional two years of training for those who want more extensive study.

Although the training program at Indore is intended to train young women to carry on KGNMT health projects, many of the trainees do not return to the local projects afterwards. Because of this, and also because Bela felt a need for the health workers to be trained on a more basic level that would offset the lack of even the most elementary health care in some of the remote projects in Orissa, she wanted to establish a local training program. In keeping with the kind of training she had done at Barpali Village Service and Mitraniketan, and even earlier when she had worked with Lies Gompertz and Joan Court in Calcutta, Bela felt that a short general purpose health training program for women who would stay with the Trust projects in Orissa would help to fill the gap.

The short course also allows women who want to receive additional training in the longer course at Indore to be working in Orissa under the supervision of a trained midwife until their turn comes.

In addition to the health worker training, the doctor generally sees only patients who come to the center, although she goes for deliveries when she is called and occasionally makes visits to homes. The health workers spend three or four afternoons each week in the nearby villages, mostly visiting prenatal and postnatal cases. If there is need for a patient to see the doctor, the health workers advise the person to go to the center.

The girls in the orphanage come from other districts of the state, being referred to the Kasturba Trust by people who are aware of the need; often the other KGNMT centers' social service workers send them. Some of the orphan girls had lived at Satyabhamapur for 10 or 12 years when I visited the project. Four or five had come that year, Bela told me. Some of the girls came because their parents could not afford to feed them; it was not always that the parents had died. Bela said that generally there are few problems with adjustment, because other children are there.

Bela knew all of the orphan children by name. The other staff members at the Kasturba Trust said that not only was Bela the KGNMT administrator, but she showed constant personal concern for the orphan girls. "She looks after their health, their clothing needs, whether they are going to school, their education," Dr. Tungavidya told me. "If they feel at all sick, she sits by their side. Though they have everybody around them, she will go and see that they get medicine."

In telling me about the orphans, Bela said. "They work very hard, these girls. They cook their food. They do their study. And then they look after all the garden. And cleaning every day. I think they work really very hard."

Although generally Bela did not enjoy her responsibility to ask for funds for the KGNMT, when it came to a project that she felt would help the orphan girls, she was eager to raise the money. At the time of my visit to the Satyabhamapur project, Bela was hoping to meet a member of the British OXFAM organization who had recently been assigned to the area. She was hoping that OXFAM would be interested in providing a tube well and a small water tower so that they could have tap water for drinking and for irrigation of the garden. "If they could have tap water, it would be much easier," she said.

Another aspect of the Satyabhamapur project in which Bela was especially interested was the nursery school which provided a pre-school education for approximately 50 children, including children from the village as well as the orphanage. Soon after she began to work at Satyabhamapur she applied for and received a grant for a new building which she described as "a proper place for the nursery school." She was hoping to convince the teachers to help the children grow a small garden beside the nursery school.

Another program Bela had started at Satyabhamapur was designed to train widows or women whose husbands had left them and who were without marketable skills. Bela was flexible in allowing women who had never married into the program as well, if they met her criteria of being destitute.

The series of six-month training programs were financed by the Orissa government who had requested the Kasturba Trust to develop the training to improve women's employment prospects. During the training the women learn to sew dresses, to embroider, and to crochet heavy, sturdy plastic bags that sell better and last longer than the traditional woven straw bags. Three classes, each of 30 or more women, had completed their training and a fourth group was being selected when I visited the KGNMT project. Members of the first two groups had received sewing machines from the government at the conclusion of their training.

Bela herself was not involved directly with the training programs at Satyabhamapur. Instead, in her role as *pratinidhi* she spent time overseeing the projects there and in each of the other nine centers in Orissa. Each of the centers had a person in charge on a day-to-day basis.

Bela's effectiveness was recognized at the national level of the Kasturba Trust. Laksmi Menon, a leader in the Indian independence movement and now chairman of the trustees of the KGNMT, talked to me about Bela when we visited in her home in Trivandrum in the state of Kerala. "In Orissa we do not have other persons like Bela. She's beginning new projects, getting help from government. We have other intense workers who are good, very practical, accommodating; they know their neighbors, but they don't get enough contacts with the outside world. And it is sure that nothing grows, if it doesn't get contact with the outside world—if it doesn't get sunlight and fresh air."

Bela's responsibility as *pratinidhi* included participation in the KGNMT annual All India Women's Conferences. The first one that she attended was in December 1979 at Poona, near Wardha. One of the speakers was the Gandhian land reform leader, Vinoba Bhave, whose *ashram* was the location for the conference. Other speakers included Bela's friends Marjorie Sykes and Laksmi Menon. Bela liked the idea of having a gathering to get to know other people, but she sensed an exaggeration in the reports of some of the *pratinidhis* when they described the work of the KGNMT centers in their states. She was troubled to learn later that failures had not been reported.

At Satyabhamapur, Dr. Tungavidya talked about Bela's role as *pratinidhi*. "As *pratinidhi* she should do the administration. But Beladi is so keen she will do from top to bottom. She will go and do everything. She is so much interested, and all-round she is. Orphanage, maternity, training program—she organizes our work and she looks after everybody's health. She is interested in each person individually; she goes and asks about them—workers in the center, children in the orphanage." The doctor continued, "She is as a younger sister to me."

Golak, the only man to work at the KGNMT office, agreed, describing Bela's activities as supervision and guidance. "She is in charge—*pratinidhi* of the institution. But she is sister to others on the staff; the orphanage girls treat her as their mother. Whenever any person faces any difficult moment she helps as much as she is able," Golak said.

Golak told me Bela had loaned him money to rebuild his house when it had been destroyed by a cyclone. Bela interrupted to give her own version of the incident. "When he went home, there was his old mother, his wife and children, but the whole house was gone. Nothing was left. Everything blown away. And he said, 'I have nothing. Everything gone. Food. Rice. Clothing. Children's books.' All was gone, so I just helped him a little bit. I gave him some money to buy some things. I didn't do much. I helped some, but I felt bad more than I helped, really."

As *pratinidhi* of the Orissa Kasturba Trust, Bela visited the ten Trust projects in the state annually. On her first visit to most of the projects in August and September 1980, a zonal organizer from the Kasturbagram head office of the Trust accompanied her. Bela was most impressed by the work at two centers in tribal areas of Koraput District. They reached one project by walking seven or eight miles up a hill. They stayed there for two days to visit a leprosy center, a nursery school and a maternity center. To get to another project, where there was also a maternity center and a nursery school, they traveled by bus, cycle rickshaw, river boat, and finally on foot, walking the last five miles. Bela explained the remote locations of the Trust projects: "Gandhiji's idea was to work with women and children in places where no doctor goes, and also to work with tribal people, against exploitation of them, and against untouchability."

Bela was impressed with both the scenery and the people at the projects in the Koraput district. "It is a beautiful place, very pleasant weather always and a natural view all round. Our worker is doing very good work with tribal people," she said.

I went with Bela to visit the Dhama-Bargoan Kasturba Trust project in Sambalpur District. Golak Chandra Das, the Orissa KGNMT accountant, and Prabha-nony Das, an influential older Gandhian worker who began the Dhama-Bargoan project in 1945 accompanied us there from Sambalpur in a jeep-taxi that they hired to take us to the project. After we got as far as the jeep could go on the narrow roads, we had a long walk through the village to reach the project on the extreme edge of the village. The next day on our return trip we walked about three miles to get back to the highway where we waited at the bus stop to catch a ride back to Sambalpur.

At the time of our visit Bela was trying to help settle a land ownership controversy. Another person had laid claim to a small amount of land where half of the well and part of a storage shed were located. Bela and Golak held meetings with the two parties involved in the dispute.

The Kasturba Trust Project at Dhama-Bargoan is very small—a nursery school for about 20 children and a maternity center that delivers an average of three babies a month. It is an attractive pastoral setting—a well-kept flower and vegetable garden in the central courtyard and around the outside of the main building, bordered by rice fields and village ponds.

In the morning Bela and I went for a walk around the project grounds. The gardener picked some guavas from the small orchard for us to eat.

Bela was concerned about the lack of interest in improving sanitation standards at the project. We tried to figure out whether the drinking water came from an open well at one end of the project or a small pond close to the bath house. Bela said that on an earlier trip they had insisted to her that it was okay to drink the water from the pond, because they didn't use the pond water for laundry or bathing.

Although there is no sealed pump well at the Kasturba Trust in Dhama-Bargoan, there are at least two in the village. One pump well was being used and a couple of people were waiting for their turn to use it both times that we walked past. Did the villagers have higher health standards than the project workers, or was it merely that the pump wells in the village were more convenient? Bela did not know.

While we were at the project, we attended a meeting of a village women's group that meets for singing and discussion nearly every evening at the Dhama-Bargoan project. One time the women had been video-taped, and a program of their singing was broadcast on television; Saki Mund, watching the program at Barpali and realizing it was one of the KGNMT projects for which Bela was responsible, complained to her husband, "Why didn't they show a picture of Beladi?"

Bela would like to see an educational effort combined with the evening singing sessions of the women. She said that Prabha-nony could influence the villagers to work toward better health habits if she was interested.

Bela also had goals for the nursery school at Dhama Bargoan and the other Kasturba centers. Her vision was to have the project work with young children and their mothers to establish more healthful standards for their lives until those standards become habit. As it is, the project has no educational effort for the nursery school children. Bela has tried to get them to install a latrine for the nursery, but they had not agreed. That didn't keep Bela from speaking out on the subject. When several children gathered around the women who had come to the project to meet us one morning and we learned that the children were enrolled in the nursery school, Bela began to talk to them and their mothers about how good it was to use the latrine.

It was not the first time while Bela and I had traveled together that she had taken on an informal role as a public health educator when she had found a natural opening. In Satlama earlier that week, she had also spoken about the importance of latrines when a group of curious schoolboys had collected around us. After exchanging greetings with the boys—they wanted to try out the few English phrases they had learned at school—Bela spoke to them in Oriya. "How many of you have latrines at home?" she asked. The only response was a few giggles. Bela talked about the smell of uncovered feces and the way that flies carried disease to their food. Some of the boys told Bela that there was a latrine at the school. A few of them professed to use it; others teasingly refuted their words. Bela turned to one boy, a little taller than the others, and asked his name. When he told her, she repeated it and then told him he should see that his family gets a latrine. "Will you?" she asked. Embarrassed, but seeming to enjoy the attention, the boy grinned and nodded his head. "I will come back in a year or two to see if you have a latrine," Bela joked.

While traveling, Bela took advantage of opportunities to give instruction in hygiene, nutrition, and social behavior. She commended children who did not litter by throwing peanut shells on the floor of the bus as others had been doing. She told a mother who bought milk from a vendor in a train station that if it hadn't been boiled it might give the baby dysentery. Once she asked a bicycle rickshaw driver whether he bought alcohol with the money that he earned; when he convinced her that he used it to buy food for his children, she said that was very good.

One of Bela's former health workers told me that Bela had cured her adult son of smoking—she gave him a sack of lemon drops and told him that whenever he felt like lighting a cigarette he should suck on a candy instead. "He never smoked again," the health worker said.

With her western friends, too, Bela gave advice about their health habits. To one friend who smoked, she wrote, "I was very happy to hear that you had stopped smoking, but when you said you had started again in two days, I was sad. You should stop for two years—like you did when you were in India—then you would not want to smoke again." To another friend she wrote, "I am glad that your daughter is nursing her baby. The mother's milk is best for the child."

Bela's eagerness to help people develop healthful habits has been at the heart of her work, even as early as her experiences at the Bengal Social Service League in the late 1930's. "I see that everything is done because of habit. If you want to do something that is better for the people you have to start from the very beginning. With little children you start. That is the most important," she said.

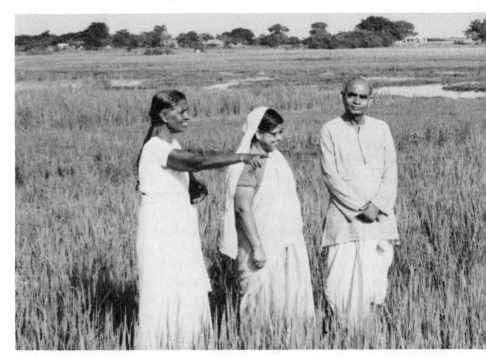

Bela with Kamala and Indubhushan Misra pointing out the paddy field which she and Kamala had chosen for the site of a "Friends Center," 1982.

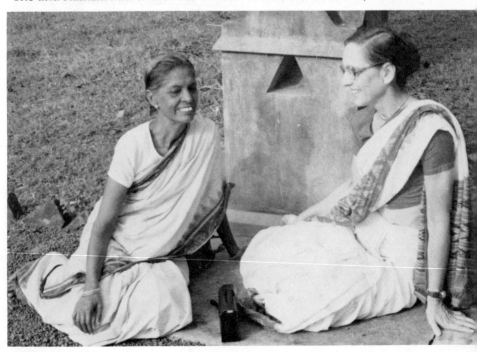

Bela and I tape-recording our conversation during our travel together in India, 1982.

PART EIGHT:

BELA'S SERVICE CONTINUES

I have had my invitation to this world's festival, and thus my life has been blessed. My eyes have seen and my ears have heard.

It was my part at this feast to play upon my instrument, and I have done all I could.

—Rabindranath Tagore
from "Gitanjali XVI"

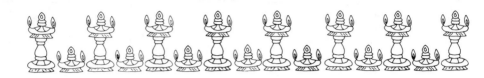

23

DREAMS FOR THE FUTURE

Bela Banerjee and I were riding in the back seat of the Mitraniketan car, her young friend Sayshee at the wheel. Maneuvering through the crowded traffic on the streets of Trivandrum with the aid of staccato beeps from the car horn, Sayshee drove out of the city and onto the scenic, curving mountain road that led to Mitraniketan.

From chatting about Bela's role as a matchmaker—she confessed to having had a part in Sayshee's choice of a wife—the conversation led to Bela's refusal of marriage when her half-brother had begun to make plans for her years before. "Instead of having nine children as you thought you didn't want, you have really been like a mother to hundreds," I said, thinking of the babies she had delivered and the many people who described her as being a mother to them. Bela laughed. "Instead of nine children, nine hundred," she said.

"I think you're not sorry for the choices you made," I suggested. "No", she agreed. "I'm happy. I'm very, very happy. Actually I was thinking I wouldn't be happy like that if I had married; I would rather be with the people."

Despite the disappointments that Bela sometimes felt in her work when others did not share her vision of what could be, she possessed an inner contentment. "Wherever I was, I always felt that this is where I should be," she told me.

Bela never sought advancement in prestige or pay or by any other yardstick with which society measures success. Yet her work, even within each project, changed and developed as she responded creatively to the needs that she perceived whenever she could help the people among whom she worked to see opportunities to improve their lives.

"Whatever I'm doing, I have faith that if I do it, it will be the right thing for me to do. If it doesn't work out for me to do it, then it wasn't right that I should do it." She paused a moment and then continued. "Each work that I have done, I have thought I would do it all my life. I never thought I would change. But as time comes, it changes, and each time, wherever I go, I feel the same way. I am always quite happy."

Even when Bela had little money and no savings, she was content. "Life was not easy, but I was not troubled by it." She looks to the future with the same assurances. "Somehow I will be managing. Something will happen; that I feel."

She is not, however, blindly optimistic in her view of the future. When someone told her that surely she would be looked after, because she had done much good work for others, she responded. "No, lots of people have done good works but have suffered much. It might come to me also. I'm ready for that. If I have to suffer, I should suffer. I'm not worried about it."

From the time she left Satish's home as a teenager to work at the Bengal Social Service League so that she could help provide for her mother, Bela exhibited characteristics of independence and courage. Remarking on these qualities, the daughter of one of the American doctors who worked with Bela at the AFSC project in Barpali, told about her memories of Bela. "It was unusual, especially in India, to be around an unmarried woman, a woman who functioned in a leadership role and who followed a life of service rather than of home and family," she said. "I think she is a kind of saint in the world, quietly going about serving others and living out her ideals."

Bela's niece Pushbanjali described Bela's response to the needs of others. "When she does something for somebody, for the moment she will forget the world. She will do and endure all sorts of things to do something for you."

At several times in her life Bela was encouraged by others to use her skills in different settings. After she left Mitraniketan in 1977, she explored a number of these opportunities.

Friends in South India invited her to work in a flood relief project they had begun when British Quakers sent money in the aftermath of a severe flood in the south Indian state of Andhra Pradesh. Because many other organizations were providing temporary direct relief to the flood victims, the couple who received the money decided to do something of a permanent nature. After designing and building six low cost houses in the area along the border of Andhra Pradesh and Madras, they invited Bela to start a clinic and form a health education center. "I wish it was in Bengal or Orissa," Bela said. But she agreed to look at the site when she went to see Viswan, who had repeatedly invited her to return to Mitraniketan to visit them at least, if not to work.

Bela described the Andhra project in a letter to Eleanor Eaton. "It is in a fishermen's village called 'Ramopuram,' a two-hour bus journey from Madras city." Bela's indecision was evident in her letter. "I wish some of you were here to see the project site. I feel it is again very far from family and friends in Calcutta, and the language is not very easy. So it is really a problem what to do," she told Eleanor. Eventually she decided not to take the position.

Dhirendranath Mund expressed a desire that Bela return to Barpali to work in public health education. Concerned about recent increases in the prevalence of leprosy in the villages near Barpali, Dr. Mund saw a role for Bela to develop a community education program so that people would not hide the disease for fear of being driven away from their homes. He said that even though effective treatment is available that can shorten the contagious period of leprosy considerably, people wait to seek treatment until their cases are so advanced that they can no longer hide the condition. By that time they may have spread the disease to others; Dr. Mund suspects that in some villages near Barpali 90 percent of the adults have leprosy.

"Unless there is an educational campaign to convince villagers to seek early treatment and to stop ostracizing people with leprosy, the condition will only continue to worsen", Dr. Mund said. Because of Bela's rapport with the villagers of the area, he believes that she would be effective in such a program. He thinks that they will listen to her when they won't listen to someone else. "She has an approach, a way of talking, that makes a difference," he said. "I think she would be a good health educator in leprosy education."

Although Bela did not see a role for herself in a leprosy education program, she remembered the leprosy treatment at BVS as having had some of the characteristics of the type of education Dr. Mund was envisioning. "At Barpali Village Service we gave leprosy patients faith," she said, remembering a time when villagers had come for treatment instead of trying to hide their disease, because they had realized they could continue to live at home.

When Bela was offered a well-paying job in a Calcutta hospital, she was not interested. "What would I do with so much money?" she said. "I would not be able to work among villagers or with the poor, as I have done all my life."

To Bela, the uncertainty of not knowing where to go for the next job, or of not always being sure that she was where she wanted to work were considerations of the moment, but not problems in planning her future. "I didn't worry at all about what would happen to me if I leave a place."

Except to the extent that she has felt the need to earn money to help others, Bela has never sought financial benefits for her work. During the time she was working at Mitraniketan, payment for her salary was provided by Community Services in Yellow Springs, Ohio, and later by the Friends Medical Society. The Friends Medical Society continued to support her financially when she worked at the Haridaspur *Seva Samiti* under a voluntary service arrangement and to some degree at Satyabhamapur where the compensation for her work as *pratinidhi* was a stipend for living expenses only. Matt Thomson, one of the American Friends Service Committee directors at Barpali Village Service, had set up an insurance fund for Bela which she recently transferred to a savings account. That small savings fund appeared to be Bela's only hedge against the future when she no longer can work.

Once at Mitraniketan Dr. Kohler had voiced the concern that others of Bela's friends have shared. "When you get old, what will you do?" Dr. Kohler had asked.

"I never thought about it and I am not worried about it," Bela responded. "Something will happen. I will manage somehow. I am very thankful that I haven't had to worry."

From the time Bela left Barpali Village Service near the close of the project in 1962, she has thought of joining with one of her health workers to set up their own maternal and child health clinic for villagers or other people who were too poor to afford doctors. At the close of BVS, village leaders came to her with a petition, asking her to set up a maternal and child health clinic which the village would finance. Despite the fact that she did not accept their invitation, the seed that they planted sprouted from time to time as Bela faced several work choices in the years that followed.

The dream draws from many sources. She thinks of the mothers and children that came to the Bengal Social Service League where she and Lies worked together in the years before independence. And she decides her dream project should be for mothers and their preschool children. She thinks of the hundreds, perhaps thousands, of babies she has delivered since the days she worked with Joan Court in

Calcutta's slums, and she wants to help to ensure healthy deliveries of newborn babies.

From the Quaker team with which she was first associated as she worked with Joan came the appeal of an adult education program that includes intellectual and cultural interchange, as well as instruction in better health habits. The training of health workers that she began at the Barpali project is a part of the dream, although now she would do it on a small scale and only train women who would plan to continue to work with her. The latrine education that was stimulated by her experiences at Barpali and developed in her work with children and women at Mitraniketan, as well as the family planning education that she initiated at Mitraniketan would be important to the center. To develop her own center would give Bela an opportunity to carry out a program of nursery school education such as she has envisioned for the Kasturba Gandhi projects. "Gandhiji said if you want peace in the world you have to start with the children," Bela says. To implement that ideal in a way that she has never seen developed is her dream.

Often when Bela has considered the possibility of beginning a project of her own, she has included Kamala Misra in her plans. They worked well together at Barpali, and have continued a close friendship through the years.

For several years Bela and Kamala dreamed of a maternal and child health center. Together they purchased a plot of ground near the village of Chawkniswanee, close to Bhubaneswar; there they hoped to build a center where they could develop a health education program around a nursery school and a clinic for women and children. Indu Misra, already involved in developing educational materials for both nursery schools and adult education literacy programs for women, would be able to work with the two women. Sarat Kanungo, who also worked with Bela at BVS and now is in charge of Government of Orissa village worker training programs, was also interested in helping to facilitate the project.

Together with Indu and Kamala Misra, Bela and I took an early morning train from Bhubaneswar to visit Bela and Kamala's plot of land. After we got off the train at Mancheswar, the station closest to Chawkniswanee, we walked past a rock crusher plant and a cement factory. Beside the factory were a stack of latrine slabs. Bela suggested that she could help them promote their product; then we noticed that the design did not include a water-seal feature that is essential to the sanitary style of latrine that she advocates. "The wrong kind," Bela said.

We walked through scrub jungle, then up a hill to a road that paralleled an irrigation canal. As we walked along, Kamala Misra pointed out the wide expanses of land and water on either side of the road. "*Sundara*, (Beautiful)," she said. We crossed the canal on a concrete beam to the other side and followed *bundhs* (dikes) between paddy fields and paths through scrub jungle to reach Bela and Kamala's small plot of ground.

It was planted to rice; the boundaries of the plot were outlined with *bundhs*. We stood in the paddy field. Bela and Kamala described their plan for the small center, showing where the building would be and anticipating their contacts with the village women and children to begin the project which Bela wants to call "Friends Center." Both women became more and more animated as they described their dream to me in ever greater detail.

Bela wants to build a center with one large room, a small room for medicine and another for her bedroom. "We would have a pump well and latrines," Bela said. She said that if other people wanted to develop an educational or agricultural aspect to the project, they could also work with her.

A few days before, Bela had laughed as she recalled a *sadhu* (Hindu holy man) who, angered because she had not given him free treatment for an infection, had once said to her, "You will be cursed never to be advanced from village work to work in the city." Watching her excitement at the plans she was envisioning for a new project in this most remote of all the places we had visited, I understood why she had seen the *sadhu's* intended curse as a blessing.

On the way back to Bhubaneswar later in the morning, Bela was quiet as we rode along on the train. We had nearly completed six weeks of travel together. I had delved into memories that had long lain dormant in her mind. She had introduced me to many of the people whose lives had intertwined with hers, and she had told me of many others. Together we had uncovered some of her roots, explored her beginnings, reviewed her life experiences, and imagined her future.

Finally she spoke in words that she intended to be a statement about her plans for the Friends Center she dreams of starting, but which seemed to me also to be a summary of a motivating force in her life. However the dream is finally realized—whether in rural Orissa, the slums of Calcutta, or some other place of need—the purpose of her life remains constant. "I want to go to the people more," she said. "I can do something that is really useful."

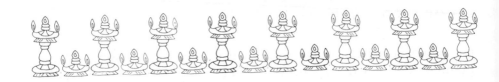

EPILOGUE

Five years have passed since I traveled with Bela and collected the material to tell her story. Her life continues to be of service to others. The dream remains, though how it will materialize still is not clear.

She and Kamala Misra found it necessary to sell the land near Bhubaneswar where they had hoped to build a health center. In 1983 she left Satyabhamapur to be an adviser for a year at an Orissa government project which was partially funded by UNICEF. She again explored possibilities to set up a private maternal and child health center in Calcutta, but like earlier attempts, the plan did not materialize because of lack of housing for the project. For most of the time since leaving the government project, she has worked again at the *Seva Samiti* project near Haridaspur, returning to help Rhomba-devi in her work among the tribal people of eastern Orissa. Now, as I write this in December 1987, Bela is in West Bengal, caring for her older sister Sushama.

Bela's life from the beginning has been one of service to others. A strong sense of family responsibilities, a profound caring for the poor, and a deep feeling of identification with other people have shaped her life and continues to give her direction.

Once Bela said to me about the poet Rabindranath Tagore, "He knew the life of the poor people so well. What really happens, he knew." Bela knows, too. Wherever she is led in the future, that knowledge will be her guide.

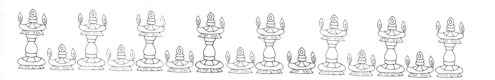

GLOSSARY

Bengali—the language spoken in West Bengal and Bangladesh
Bhagavad Gita—one of the books of Hindu scripture
bai—term used for one's mother or highly respected older woman
bhai—brother (used as a suffix to a person's name)
Brahman—person of the priestly caste of Hindus
Brahmo Samaj—religious reform group growing out of Hinduism in the mid-19th
    century
bundhs—dikes or ridges separating paddy fields, used as paths
burkha—outer garment covering head to foot, worn by Muslim women
bustee—slum area
chai—Indian tea made with milk and sugar
chai walla—vendor who sells Indian tea in train stations
chappals—Indian sandals with no ties or buckles, easily removed
chappaties—unleavened bread rolled into flat circles, cooked on a hot griddle
charpoy—a village cot of woven rope on a wooden frame
chechi—sister (Malayalam)
chhordi—little sister (Bengali)
chula—stove made of clay, usually built low just off the earthen floor in an Indian
    kitchen
devi—a term of respect attached as a suffix to a woman's name
dhal—lentils cooked with spices and served with rice
didi—sister (used as a title or as a suffix to a person's name)
Durga Puja—Hindu holiday held in the autumn
guru—teacher, spiritual leader
Harijan—untouchable, lowest position within Hinduism
Hindi—a north Indian language, now national language of India
Hindu—a person who practices the religion of Hinduism
Malayalam—the language spoken in Kerala
muri—puffed rice eaten as a snack
namaskar, namaste—words used for greetings in much of India
Oriya—the language spoken in Orissa
pratinidhi—administrator or director
purdah—seclusion of Moslem women behind a veil or a *burkah* when in public
rupees—Indian currency (has ranged from 3 to 12.5 rupees to the U.S. dollar in the last
    40 years)
sari—traditional garment worn by women in most parts of India
sujee—a porridge similar to cream-of-wheat
zamindar—a landlord who collected taxes and other revenue under British rule
zamindari—the land owned or controlled by a zamindar

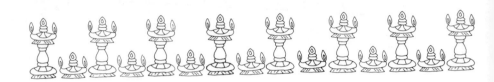

INDEX